HEMODYNAMIC WAVEFORMS

Exercises in identification and analysis

To the
critical care specialists
who provide the essential link in patient care in
coronary care units and intensive care units
throughout the world

HEMODYNAMIC WAVEFORMS
Exercises in identification and analysis

ELAINE KIESS DAILY, R.N., B.S., R.C.V.T.

Cardiovascular Nurse Specialist,
Consultant, and Lecturer,
Palo Alto, California

JOHN SPEER SCHROEDER, M.D.

Director, Coronary Care Unit, and
Associate Professor of Clinical Medicine,
Stanford University Medical Center,
Stanford, California

with **199** illustrations

The C. V. Mosby Company

ST. LOUIS · TORONTO · LONDON   1983

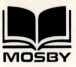

MOSBY

A TRADITION OF PUBLISHING EXCELLENCE

Editor: Michael R. Riley
Assistant editor: Sally Gaines
Manuscript editor: Marjorie L. Sanson
Book design: Jeanne Bush
Cover design: Suzanne Oberholtzer
Production: Barbara Merritt

The C.V. Mosby Company
11830 Westline Industrial Drive, St. Louis, Missouri 63141

Library of Congress Cataloging in Publication Data

Daily, Elaine Kiess.
    Hemodynamic waveforms.

    Bibliography: p.
    1. Hemodynamics—Problems, exercises, etc.
2. Patient monitoring—Problems, exercises, etc.
I. Schroeder, John Speer, 1937-   II. Title.
[DNLM: 1. Critical care—Nursing texts. 2. Coronary care units—Nursing texts. 3. Hemodynamics—Nursing texts. 4. Monitoring, Physiologic—Nursing texts. WY 152.5.D133h]
QP105.D34   1983   616.07'54   82-12419
ISBN 0-8016-1212-8

C/VH/VH   9 8 7 6 5 4 3 2 1   01/A/041

Preface

Our experience lecturing to critical care nurses and specialists throughout the United States has made us acutely aware of the need for practical experience in identifying and interpreting hemodynamic waveforms. Thus the purpose of this book is to provide this experience by presenting the opportunity to study a variety of hemodynamic pressure waveforms. It is hoped that this book will serve as a detailed supplement to our *Techniques in Bedside Hemodynamic Monitoring* (1981, The C.V. Mosby Co.), which provides basic discussion, information, guidelines, and techniques. It is intended for the individual who has a solid foundation in the physiology and techniques of hemodynamic monitoring and who is now ready for more intense, practical learning experiences. Those pressure waveforms that appear in *Techniques in Bedside Hemodynamic Monitoring* are primarily ideal, normal tracings selected to teach the physiologic events responsible for the pressure changes. Unfortunately, the ideal, normal pressure tracing is seldom encountered in the clinical situation. Although they are necessary and useful to teach the basic principles of hemodynamic monitoring, they are not always practical. This book, then, expands on the reader's basic knowledge and offers a variety of actual pressure tracings of the type encountered in the clinical setting.

The first five chapters review the physiologic events that produce specific hemodynamic waveforms, as well as their correlation to the ECG and causes of commonly seen abnormalities. Following the discussions are examples of numerous, varied normal and abnormal hemodynamic waveforms with analysis and pertinent comments. Chapter six includes case studies of individual patients to illustrate the hemodynamic abnormalities in certain disorders and their response to specific therapies. The last chapter is a self-assessment section in which the reader is asked to exercise skills in identification and analysis of numerous hemodynamic waveforms. One correct interpretation is on the reverse side of the page for immediate reinforcement or correction. Many of the hemodynamic waveforms throughout this book could be seen in more than one pathologic condition. To enhance learning and avoid the confusion of a long list of possible causes, we have listed only the most likely pathologic condition. Needless to say, the experienced hemodynamicist could determine other, equally correct causes of the abnormality.

We have been promising a workbook to critical care nurses and physicians throughout the United States for over a year, with the hope that it will lead to a greater understanding of the physiologic causes of hemodynamic pressure waveforms, improve identification and interpretation skills, and thereby ease the problems that all too often are associated with hemodynamic monitoring.

Special acknowledgment must be accorded Dr. E.W. Hancock for kindly reviewing a number of troublesome pressure tracings. Both his time and input are greatly appreciated. We are also grateful to Mrs. Mary Lou Guerriere for so promptly and correctly typing this manuscript. Elaine Daily wishes to thank her parents for taking over so many of her other responsibilities from time to time so that work on this book could continue.

Elaine Kiess Daily
John Speer Schroeder

Contents

Abbreviations

APC	Atrial premature contraction
BPM	Beats per minute
CI	Cardiac index
CO	Cardiac output
FA	Femoral artery
LA	Left atrium
LAD	Left anterior descending
LV	Left ventricle
LVedp	Left ventricular end-diastolic pressure
LVH	Left ventricular hypertrophy
MI	Myocardial infarction or mitral insufficiency
PA	Pulmonary artery
PAedp	Pulmonary artery end-diastolic pressure
PAW	Pulmonary artery wedge
PNB	Premature nodal beat
PVC	Premature ventricular contraction
PVR	Pulmonary vascular resistance
RA	Right atrium
RV	Right ventricle
RVedp	Right ventricular end-diastolic pressure
SVR	Systemic vascular resistance
VT	Ventricular tachycardia

Normal values

RA (*a/v*/mean)	8/8/2-6 mm Hg
RV (sys/dias/end-dias)	20-30/0-5/2-6 mm Hg
PA (sys/dias/mean)	20-30/10-15/10-20 mm Hg
PAW (*a/v*/mean)	12-15/12-15/4-12 mm Hg
LA (*a/v*/mean)	12-15/12-15/4-12 mm Hg
LV (sys/dias/end-dias)	100-140/0-5/5-12 mm Hg
Arterial (sys/dias/mean)	100-140/60-80/70 mm Hg
Cardiac output	4.0-8.0 L/min
Cardiac index	2.5-4.0 L/min/m^2
Stroke volume	60-130 ml/beat
Systemic vascular resistance	15-20 units or 900-1600 dynes/sec/cm^{-5}

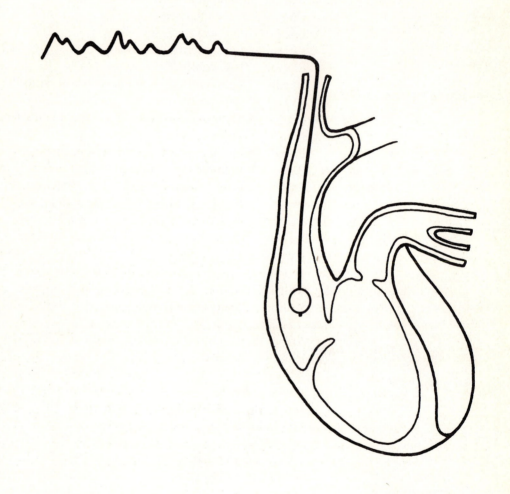

chapter 1

Right atrial pressures

Physiology and morphology

The pressure changes produced by the right atrium are small and usually consist of three distinct positive waves—*a, c,* and *v*—followed by negative waves—*x, x*^{1}*,* and *y* descents. The *a* wave is a small pressure rise that is produced by the action of atrial systole. The decline in pressure that immediately follows the *a* wave is termed the *x* descent and reflects a decrease in right atrial volume during atrial relaxation (immediately following systole). The *c* wave may appear as a distinct wave, as a notch on the *a* wave, or may be absent altogether. It reflects a slight increase in pressure in the right atrium produced by closure of the tricuspid valve leaflets. The negative wave immediately following the *c* wave is termed the *x*^{1} descent. It is produced by a downward pulling of the septum during ventricular systole. (If the *c* wave appears only as notch on the *a* wave, the single descent following the *ac* wave is termed the *x* descent.)

The *v* wave is an increase in atrial pressure produced by right atrial filling and concomitant right ventricular systole, which causes the leaflets of the closed tricuspid valve to actually bulge back into the right atrium. The *y* descent immediately follows the *v* wave and is produced by the opening of the tricuspid valve and emptying of the right atrium into the right ventricle.

Since the pressure rises produced during both the atrial systolic (*a* wave) and diastolic (*v* wave) events are nearly the same (usually within 3 to 4 mm Hg of each other), we generally take an average or a mean of the pressure rises. The normal resting mean right atrial pressure is 2 to 6 mm Hg.

ECG correlation

The *a* wave, which represents mechanical atrial systole, immediately succeeds electrical atrial depolarization, i.e., after the P wave of the ECG. Because of the time required for the mechanical event to reach the sensing device (the transducer) and depending on the length of tubing used, there is a varying degree of delay between the recorded electrical event and the mechanical event. At any rate, the *a* wave of the atrial pressure generally is seen during the PR interval of the ECG.

The *c* wave, reflecting closure of the tricuspid valve, corresponds to the RS-T junction of the ECG.

The v wave, representing ventricular systole, would naturally succeed electrical ventricular depolarization and can be looked for any time in the TP interval.

Atrial fibrillation is characterized by the absence of uniform atrial depolarization and consequently results in absent P waves in the ECG and absent a waves in the right atrial pressure waveform. For every QRS complex, there will be one distinct pressure rise, the v wave. Frequently, however, it is possible to see small flutter or fibrillatory waves throughout the pressure tracing.

In junctional rhythm or during certain beats of AV dissociation where the atria contract against a closed tricuspid valve, giant a or cannon a waves are seen in the right atrial pressure tracing.

Patients with a ventricular pacemaker may have absent a waves, occasional, random a waves, or even cannon a waves at times. This is the result of absent or dissociated atrial activity that does not relate to the QRS.

Abnormal findings

Elevated RA pressures occur in the following cases:
1. Right ventricular failure
2. Tricuspid stenosis and regurgitation
3. Cardiac tamponade
4. Constrictive pericarditis
5. Pulmonary hypertension (primary or secondary)
6. Chronic left ventricular failure
7. Volume overload

The a wave of the RA pressure tracing is exaggerated and elevated in any condition that increases the resistance to right ventricular filling. These include tricuspid stenosis, RV failure, pulmonary hypertension, and pulmonic stenosis.

The v wave of the RA pressure tracing is exaggerated and elevated in tricuspid regurgitation due to a reflux of blood into the right atrium during ventricular systole through the insufficiently closed tricuspid valve.

In cardiac tamponade both the a and v waves are elevated and reflect the elevated diastolic filling pressures in all chambers of the heart. The contour of the RA pressure tracing is distinct, however, showing a predominant x descent with a very short or absent y descent.

In constrictive pericardial disease the a and v waves of the RA pressure tracing are also elevated, but the contour of the waveform differs from cardiac tamponade, showing either a predominant y descent or equally dominant x and y descents. Additionally, Kussmaul's sign (a rise rather than a fall in right atrial pressure during inspiration) can be seen in constrictive disease but rarely, if ever, in cardiac tamponade.

Respiratory variation is often quite marked in the RA pressure waveform. Taking an average or mean pressure throughout three respiratory cycles diminishes this problem. Recording the pressure at the end of the expiratory phase of the breathing cycle minimizes this problem.

Positive pressure mechanical ventilation elevates the measured RA pressure, reflecting the increase in intrathoracic pressure. However, the actual pressure in the RA may be reduced as a result of a decrease in venous return. Recording pressures both on and off the ventilator provides a more accurate picture of the effects of mechanical ventilation and the actual volemic state of the patient, if this can be done without severely compromising oxygenation.

Inaccurate zeroing or calibration will produce an erroneous RA pressure value and should be suspected if the RA pressure does not correlate with the clinical picture.

Placement of the air reference stopcock above the level of the RA will produce an erroneously low RA pressure, whereas placement below the RA produces an erroneously high RA pressure.

Examples

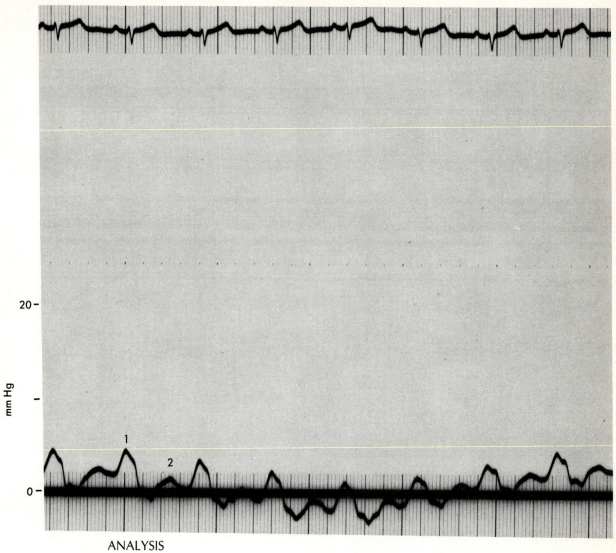

ANALYSIS

Rhythm: NSR

Pressure(s): RA

Waveform characteristics and measurements:

1. _____ *a* Wave _____ ;	5	mm Hg
2. _____ *v* Wave _____ ;	2	mm Hg
3. _____ Mean _____ ;	3	mm Hg
4. _____ ;	_____	mm Hg
5. _____ ;	_____	mm Hg
6. _____ ;	_____	mm Hg
7. _____ ;	_____	mm Hg

Suspected abnormality: Normal

Comments: Note the normal fall in atrial pressure during inspiration due to the effect of negative intrathoracic pressure.

4

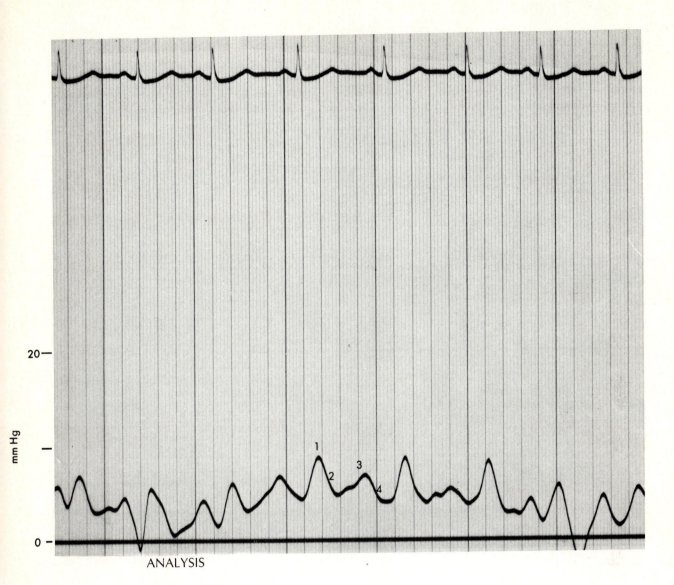

ANALYSIS

Rhythm: NSR

Pressure(s): RA

Waveform characteristics and measurements:

1.	*a* Wave	;	7	mm Hg
2.	*x* Descent	;		mm Hg
3.	*v* Wave	;	6	mm Hg
4.	*y* Descent	;		mm Hg
5.	Mean	;	5	mm Hg
6.		;		mm Hg
7.		;		mm Hg

Suspected abnormality: Normal

Comments: Note the normal respiratory variation with a fall in atrial pressure during inspiration. Note, also, the normal delay of the *a* wave following the ECG P wave.

5

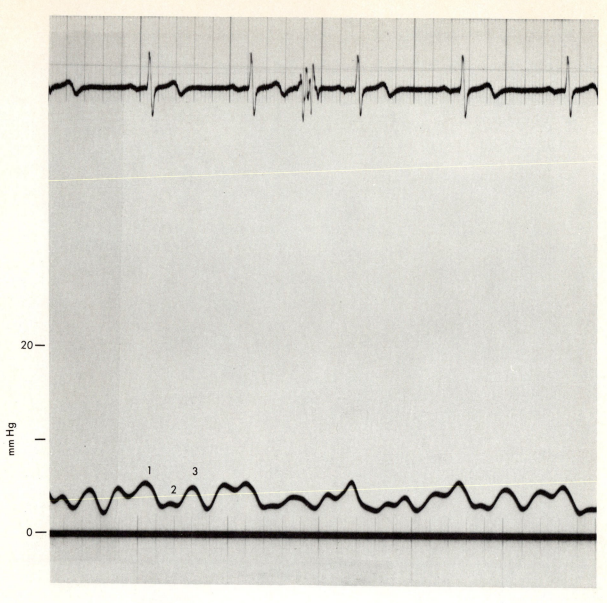

ANALYSIS

Rhythm: NSR

Pressure(s): RA

Waveform characteristics and measurements:

1.	*a* Wave	;	5	mm Hg
2.	*c* Wave	;		mm Hg
3.	*v* Wave	;	5	mm Hg
4.	Mean	;	4	mm Hg
5.		;		mm Hg
6.		;		mm Hg
7.		;		mm Hg

Suspected abnormality: Normal

Comments:

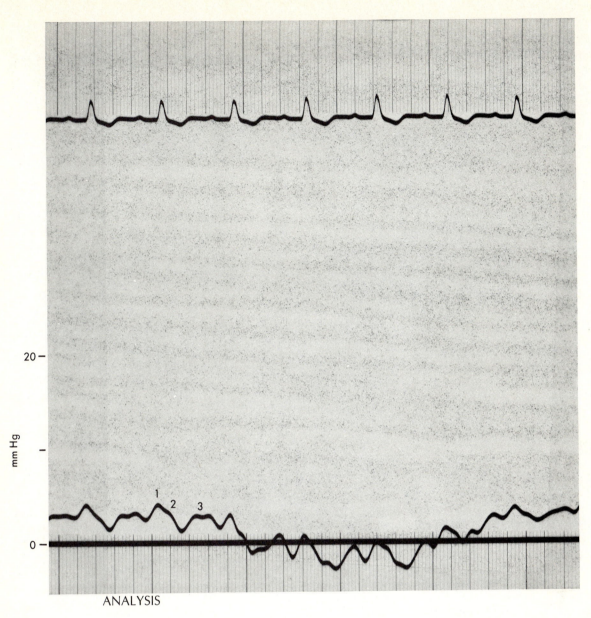

ANALYSIS

Rhythm: NSR

Pressure(s): RA

Waveform characteristics and measurements:

1.	*a* Wave	;	2	mm Hg
2.	*c* Wave	;		mm Hg
3.	*v* Wave	;	1	mm Hg
4.	Mean	;	2	mm Hg
5.		;		mm Hg
6.		;		mm Hg
7.		;		mm Hg

Suspected abnormality: Normal or hypovolemia

Comments: Note the normal respiratory response of a fall in pressure during inspiration, even to negative values.

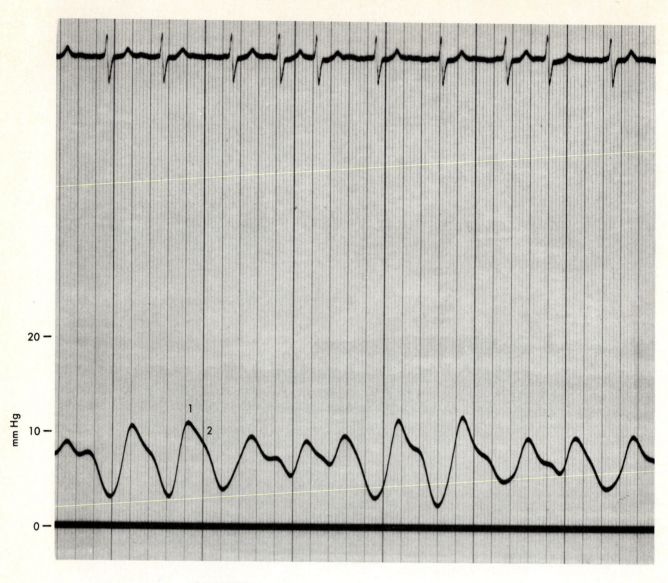

ANALYSIS

Rhythm: Atrial fibrillation

Pressure(s): RA

Waveform characteristics and measurements:

1.	*v* Wave	;	10 mm Hg
2.	*y* Descent	;	mm Hg
3.	Mean	;	8 mm Hg
4.		;	mm Hg
5.		;	mm Hg
6.		;	mm Hg
7.		;	mm Hg

Suspected abnormality: Mild RV failure

Comments: Note the effect of changing RR intervals on the extent of the *y* descent reflecting changes in duration of RV filling. The absence of an *a* wave is due to atrial fibrillation.

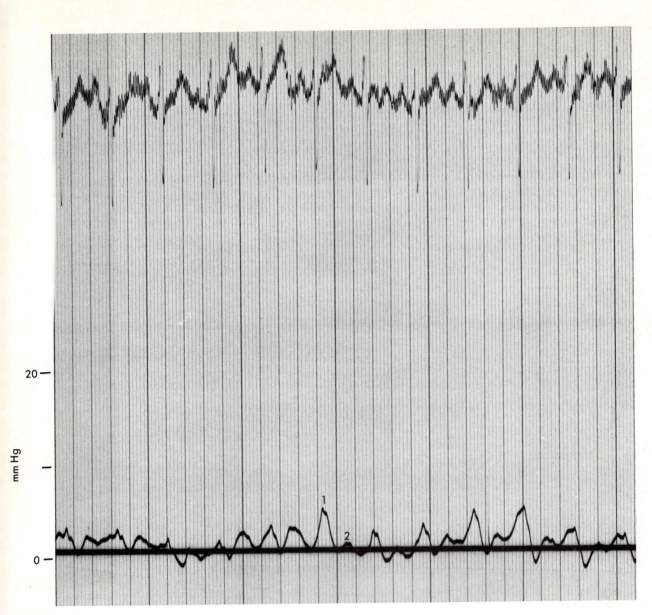

ANALYSIS

Rhythm: NSR (note 60-cycle electrical interference in ECG)

Pressure(s): RA

Waveform characteristics and measurements:

1.	*a* Wave	;	3	mm Hg
2.	*v* Wave	;	1	mm Hg
3.	Mean	;	2	mm Hg
4.		;		mm Hg
5.		;		mm Hg
6.		;		mm Hg
7.		;		mm Hg

Suspected abnormality: Hypovolemia (or normal)

Comments:

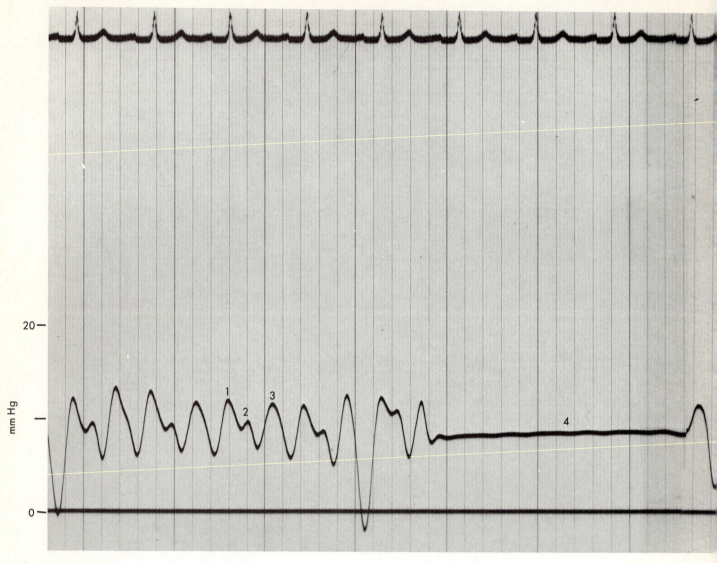

ANALYSIS

Rhythm: NSR

Pressure(s): RA

Waveform characteristics and measurements:

1.	*a* Wave	;	14	mm Hg
2.	*c* Wave	;		mm Hg
3.	*v* Wave	;	14	mm Hg
4.	Electrical mean	;	10	mm Hg
5.		;		mm Hg
6.		;		mm Hg
7.		;		mm Hg

Suspected abnormality: Hypervolemia or RV failure

Comments: Note exaggerated inspiratory response bringing the *y* descent below baseline at times.

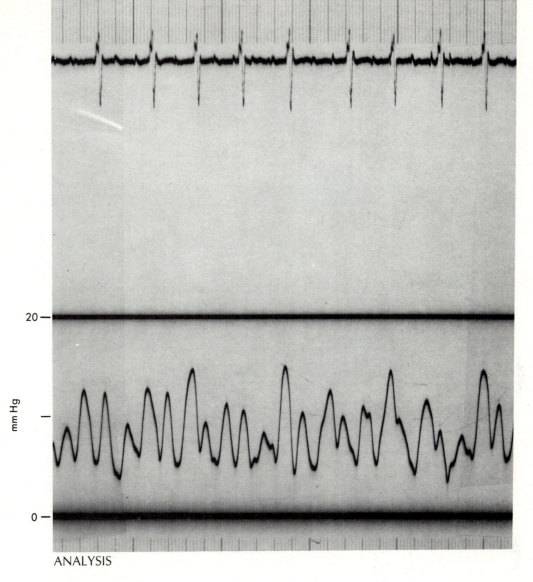

ANALYSIS

Rhythm: Probably atrial flutter with varying block

Pressure(s): RA

Waveform characteristics and measurements:

1. _____Mean_____ ; _____8_____ mm Hg
2. _____ ; _____ mm Hg
3. _____ ; _____ mm Hg
4. _____ ; _____ mm Hg
5. _____ ; _____ mm Hg
6. _____ ; _____ mm Hg
7. _____ ; _____ mm Hg

Suspected abnormality: Normal

Comments: This RA waveform displays a number of oscillations that are primarily flutter waves occasionally superimposed on small v waves.

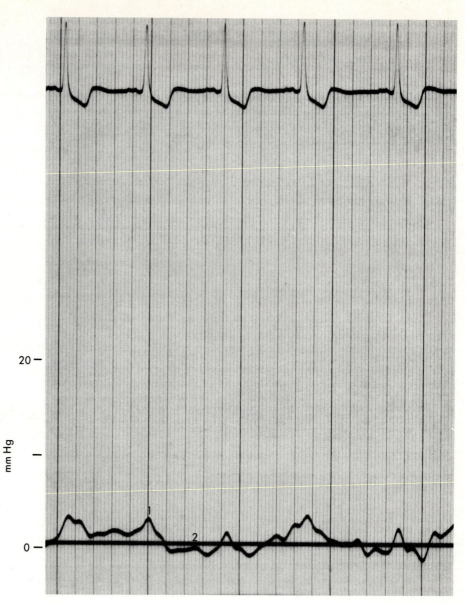

ANALYSIS

Rhythm: NSR

Pressure(s): RA

Waveform characteristics and measurements:

1.	*a* Wave	;	2	mm Hg
2.	*v* Wave	;	1	mm Hg
3.	Mean	;	1	mm Hg
4.		;		mm Hg
5.		;		mm Hg
6.		;		mm Hg
7.		;		mm Hg

Suspected abnormality: Hypovolemia secondary to diuresis

Comments:

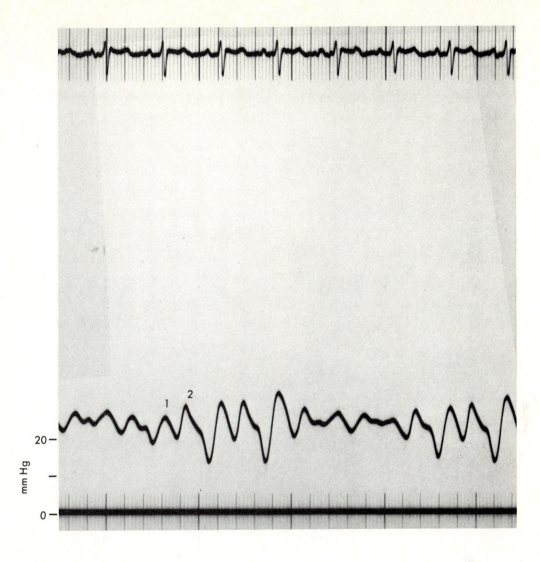

ANALYSIS

Rhythm: NSR

Pressure(s): RA

Waveform characteristics and measurements:

1.	*a* Wave	;	24	mm Hg
2.	*v* Wave	;	25	mm Hg
3.	Mean	;	21	mm Hg
4.		;		mm Hg
5.		;		mm Hg
6.		;		mm Hg
7.		;		mm Hg

Suspected abnormality: CHF

Comments: CHF of long standing is eventually reflected back as an elevation of the RA pressure. Note exaggerated *x* and *y* descents during inspiration and the minimal delay between the electrical and mechanical events with the use of a miniature transducer attached directly to the catheter.

13

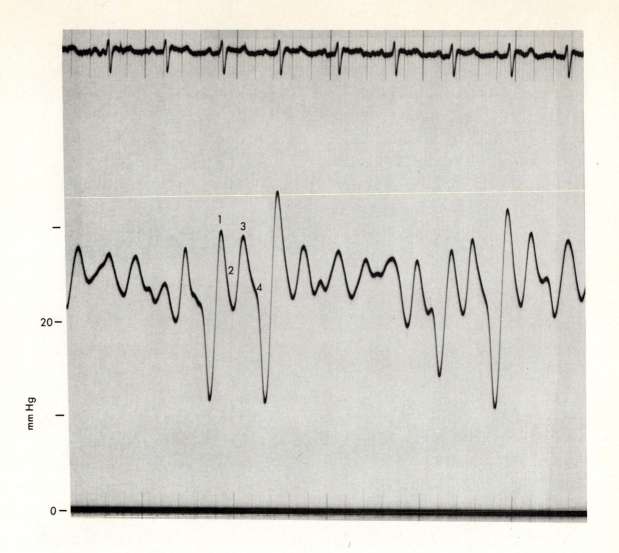

ANALYSIS

Rhythm: NSR

Pressure(s): RA

Waveform characteristics and measurements:

1.	*a* Wave	;	28	mm Hg
2.	*x* Descent	;		mm Hg
3.	*v* Wave	;	27	mm Hg
4.	*y* Descent	;		mm Hg
5.	Mean	;	25	mm Hg
6.		;		mm Hg
7.		;		mm Hg

Suspected abnormality: RV failure possibly secondary to RV infarction

Comments: Note the marked respiratory variation.

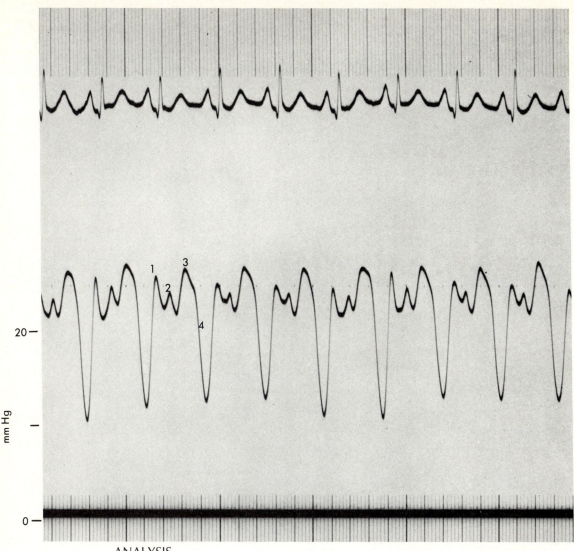

ANALYSIS

Rhythm: NSR

Pressure(s): RA

Waveform characteristics and measurements:

1.	*a* Wave	;	25	mm Hg
2.	*c* Wave	;		mm Hg
3.	*v* Wave	;	27	mm Hg
4.	*y* Descent	;		mm Hg
5.	Mean	;	19	mm Hg
6.		;		mm Hg
7.		;		mm Hg

Suspected abnormality: Constrictive pericarditis

Comments: Note the elevated *a* and *v* waves with a predominant *y* descent consistent with constrictive pericardial disease. The exaggerated *y* descent is due to rapid ventricular filling (atrial emptying) during early diastole followed by an abrupt rise in pressure as the size of the heart is increased and compressed by the inelastic, constricted pericardium.

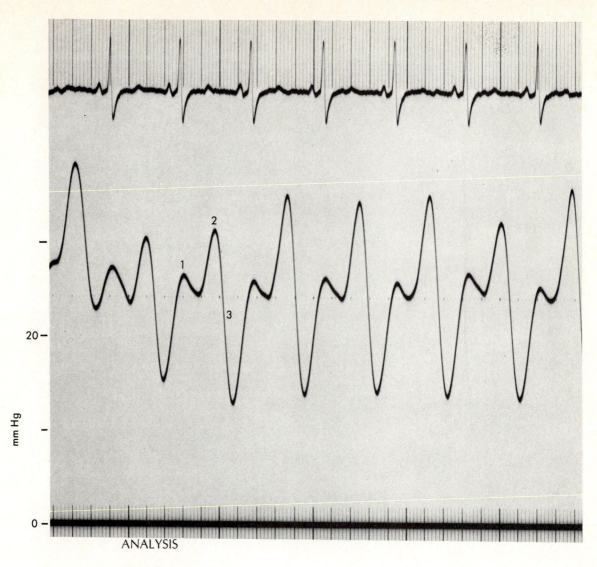

ANALYSIS

Rhythm: NSR

Pressure(s): RA

Waveform characteristics and measurements:

1.	*a* Wave	;	26	mm Hg
2.	*v* Wave	;	34	mm Hg
3.	*y* Descent	;		mm Hg
4.		;		mm Hg
5.		;		mm Hg
6.		;		mm Hg
7.		;		mm Hg

Suspected abnormality: RV Failure with tricuspid insufficiency secondary to RV infarction

Comments: Both the *a* and *v* waves of this RA waveform are elevated with a dominant *v* wave and a rapid *y* descent. This is due to tricuspid regurgitation with an increase in blood volume in the right atrium during ventricular systole. The *a* wave of 26 mm Hg reflects an elevated RVedp and RV failure. This type of hemodynamic picture can be seen in RV infarction, with dilatation of the right ventricle producing some tricuspid regurgitation.

16

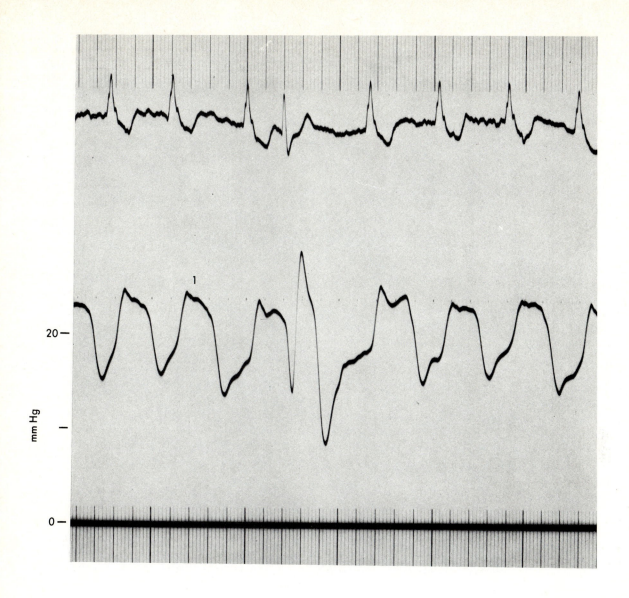

ANALYSIS

Rhythm: Atrial fibrillation with PNB

Pressure(s): RA

Waveform characteristics and measurements:

1. _____ *v* Wave _____ ; _____ 24 _____ mm Hg
2. _____ ; _____ mm Hg
3. _____ ; _____ mm Hg
4. _____ ; _____ mm Hg
5. _____ ; _____ mm Hg
6. _____ ; _____ mm Hg
7. _____ ; _____ mm Hg

Suspected abnormality: RV failure with tricuspid insufficiency secondary to RV dilatation

Comments: Note the increased *v* wave following the premature nodal beat.

17

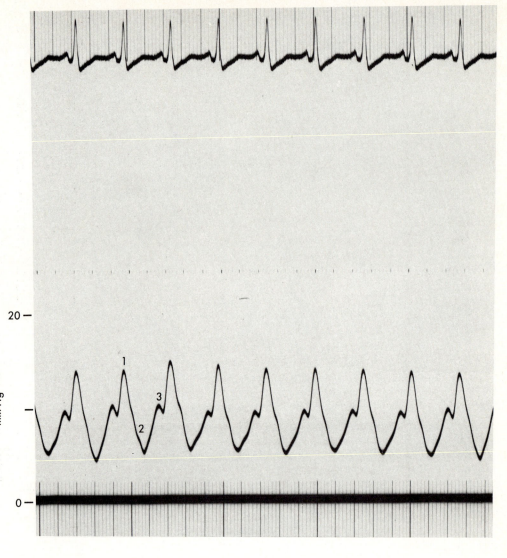

ANALYSIS

Rhythm: Sinus tachycardia

Pressure(s): RA

Waveform characteristics and measurements:

1.		*a* Wave	;	14	mm Hg
2.		*x* Descent	;		mm Hg
3.		*v* Wave	;	10	mm Hg
4.		Mean	;	10	mm Hg
5.			;		mm Hg
6.			;		mm Hg
7.			;		mm Hg

Suspected abnormality: RV failure secondary to LV failure

Comments: The dominant and elevated *a* wave suggests increased resistance to ventricular filling due to a failing, noncompliant RV.

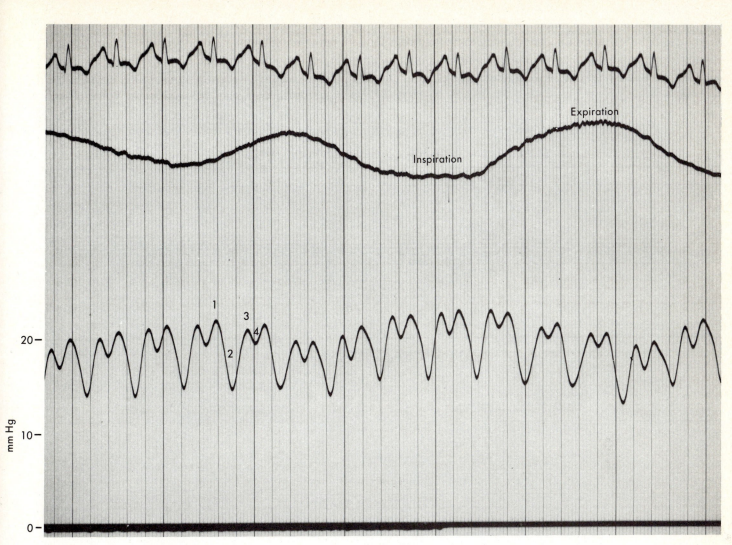

ANALYSIS

Rhythm: Sinus tachycardia

Pressure(s): RA

Waveform characteristics and measurements:

1.	*a* Wave	;	20 mm Hg
2.	*x* Descent	;	mm Hg
3.	*v* Wave	;	20 mm Hg
4.	*y* Descent	;	mm Hg
5.	Mean	;	19 mm Hg
6.		;	mm Hg
7.		;	mm Hg

Suspected abnormality: Effusive-constrictive pericardial disease

Comments: Effusive-constrictive pericarditis refers to a combined condition in which there is both visceral pericardial constriction and the presence of effusion in the pericardial space. The RA pressure is elevated as a compensatory mechanism to adequately fill the heart. The contour of the RA pressure usually discloses approximately equal *a* and *v* waves with either a prominent *x* descent (as in cardiac tamponade) or equal *x* and *y* descents. Normally the atrial pressure falls during inspiration due to negative intrathoracic pressure. Note the rise, rather than a fall, in this venous pressure during inspiration. This is termed *Kussmaul's sign* and is seen in constrictive pericardial disease and not in pericardial effusion. It is due to a failure of transmission of negative intrathoracic pressure through the rigid pericardium to the heart.

19

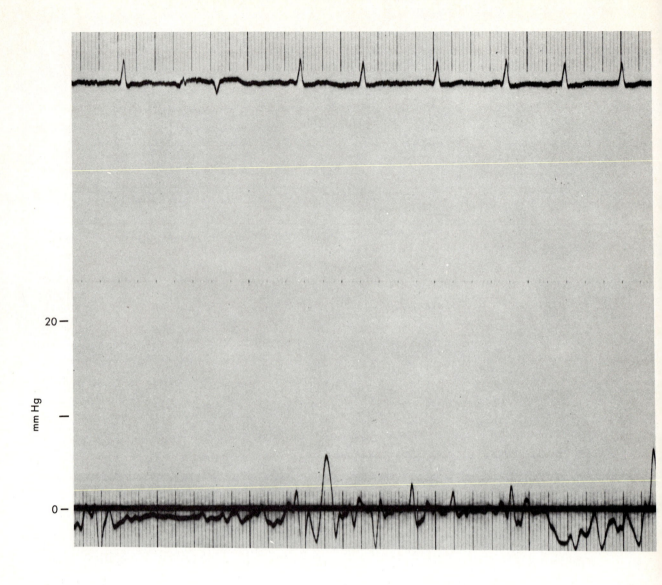

ANALYSIS

Rhythm: Atrial fibrillation

Pressure(s): (?)

Waveform characteristics and measurements:

1. _____ ; _____ mm Hg

2. _____ ; _____ mm Hg

3. _____ ; _____ mm Hg

4. _____ ; _____ mm Hg

5. _____ ; _____ mm Hg

6. _____ ; _____ mm Hg

7. _____ ; _____ mm Hg

Suspected abnormality: Improper zeroing or loose connection

Comments:

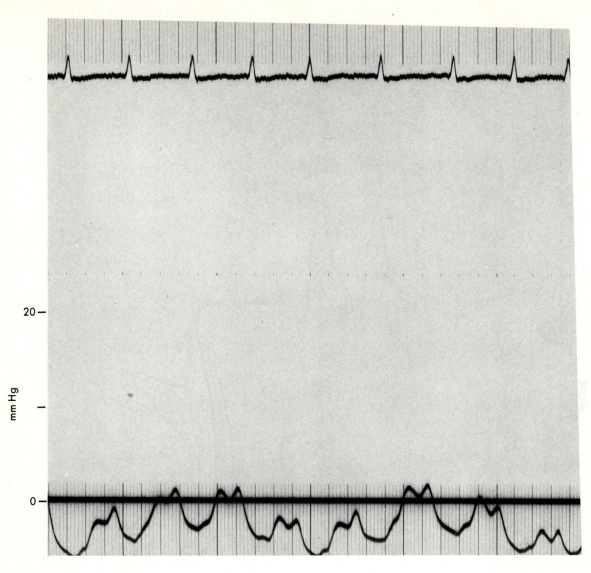

ANALYSIS

Rhythm: Atrial fibrillation

Pressure(s): (?) Possibly RA

Waveform characteristics and measurements:

1. _____ ; _____ mm Hg

2. _____ ; _____ mm Hg

3. _____ ; _____ mm Hg

4. _____ ; _____ mm Hg

5. _____ ; _____ mm Hg

6. _____ ; _____ mm Hg

7. _____ ; _____ mm Hg

Suspected abnormality: Transducer air reference level positioned above the level of the
patient's right atrium

Comments:

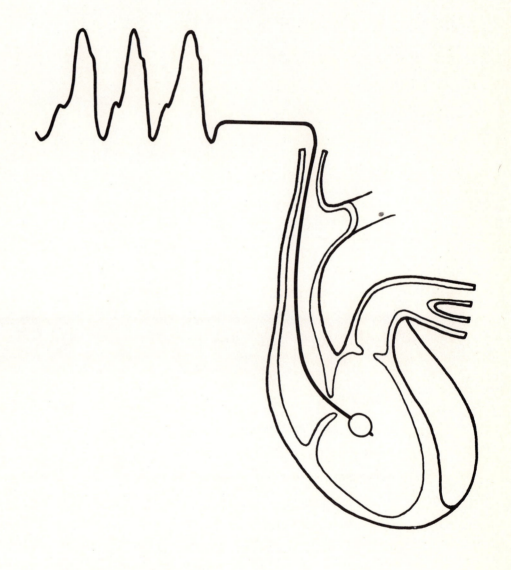

chapter 2

Right ventricular pressures

Physiology and morphology

The pressure changes in the right ventricle reflect the dynamic, pumping action of that chamber. In general, the phases are systole and diastole; however, these are broken down further into seven specific events that constitute ventricular dynamics.

Systolic events	Diastolic events
1. Isovolumetric contraction	4. Isovolumetric relaxation
2. Rapid ejection	5. Early diastole
3. Reduced ejection	6. Atrial systole (kick)
	7. End-diastole

Isovolumetric contraction refers to the increase in tension or pressure due to ventricular muscle contraction without any change in ventricular volume. ("Iso" means equal; "volumetric" refers to volume.) This is because both the tricuspid and pulmonic valves are closed during this time. The continued rise in ventricular pressure, however, forces the pulmonic valve open, and *rapid ejection* of blood into the pulmonary artery occurs. *Reduced ejection* is characterized by a drop in ventricular pressure, even though some blood is still being pumped into the PA.

Diastole occurs when the ventricular pressure has dropped lower than the PA pressure, causing the pulmonic valve to close. This sharp decline in pressure is due to *isovolumetric relaxation*. The ventricular muscle fibers are relaxing and losing tension while both pulmonic and tricuspid valves are closed, obviating any changes in ventricular volume. When the ventricular diastolic pressure falls below the RA pressure, the tricuspid valve opens, resulting in passive filling of the right ventricle. This period is termed *early diastole* or the rapid filling phase. This is soon followed by atrial systole, which forces an additional volume (anywhere from 10% to 15%) of blood into the ventricle. It is evidenced by an increase in pressure, termed the *atrial kick* or simply the *a* wave.

The period immediately succeeding the *a* wave, just before the systolic pressure rise occurs, is termed *end-diastole*. The pressure during this period reflects end-diastolic volume. It is the ventricular end-diastolic volume that determines the extent of fiber shortening and the subsequent stroke volume according to the Starling law.

ECG correlation

The systolic ejection phase corresponds to ventricular depolarization, or more generally the QT interval of the ECG. The diastolic period occurs, generally, in the TQ period of the ECG.

Abnormal findings

Elevation of the right ventricular systolic pressure occurs with pulmonary hypertension (whatever the cause), VSD, or pulmonic stenosis. Normally the RV and PA systolic pressures are essentially equal. In pulmonic stenosis the RV systolic pressure is much greater than the PA systolic pressure due to the resistance to ejection met at the narrowed pulmonic valve.

The RV diastolic pressure is elevated in right ventricular failure, constrictive pericarditis, or cardiac tamponade. Left-sided heart failure of long standing may also be reflected back as an increase in RVedp.

Right ventricular pressure is usually not directly monitored at the bedside. However, it is indirectly monitored through evaluation of the PA systolic pressure, which equals RV systolic pressure, and the RA mean pressure, which approximates the RV end-diastolic pressure (if tricuspid or pulmonic valvular disease is not present). Knowledge of the events producing the RV pressure waveform is useful, since the same physiologic events produce the left ventricular pressure. Accurate identification of RV pressure waveform is essential for safe, accurate hemodynamic monitoring. The presence of an RV pressure waveform on the oscilloscope requires withdrawal of the catheter to the RA or inflation of the balloon for flotation of the catheter out to the PA.

Examples

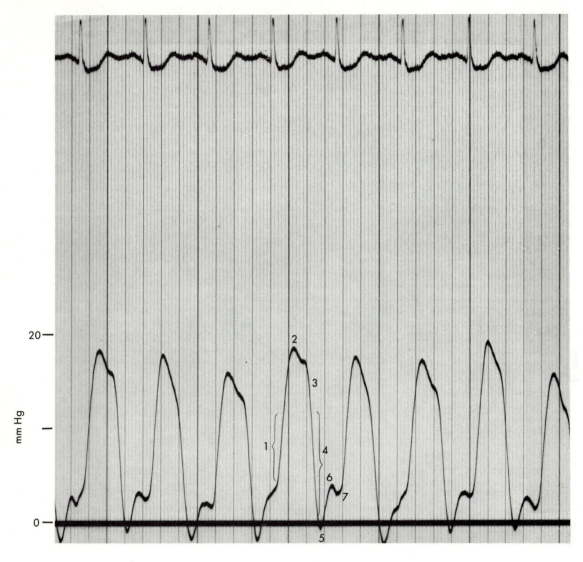

ANALYSIS

Rhythm: NSR

Pressure(s): RV

Waveform characteristics and measurements:

1.	Isovolumetric contraction	;		mm Hg
2.	Rapid ejection	;		mm Hg
3.	Reduced ejection	;		mm Hg
4.	Isovolumetric relaxation	;		mm Hg
5.	Early diastole	;		mm Hg
6.	Atrial systole	;		mm Hg
7.	End-diastole	;		mm Hg

Suspected abnormality: Normal

Comments: Note the early diastolic pressure falling to baseline and below.

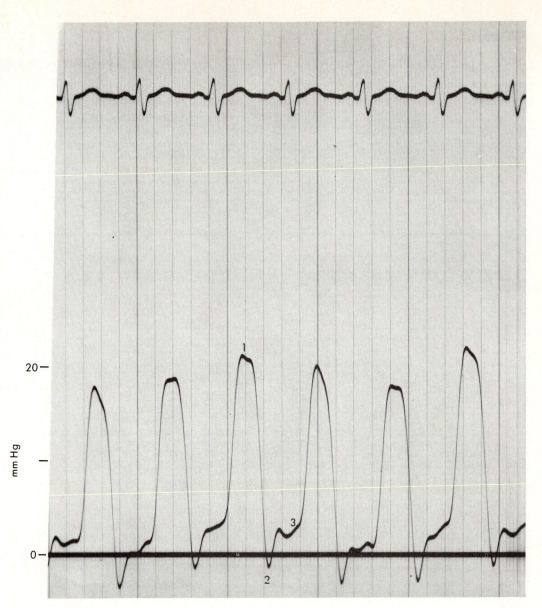

ANALYSIS

Rhythm: NSR

Pressure(s): RV

Waveform characteristics and measurements:

1.	RV systolic	;	20	mm Hg
2.	RV early diastolic dip	;		mm Hg
3.	RV end-diastolic	;	2	mm Hg
4.		;		mm Hg
5.		;		mm Hg
6.		;		mm Hg
7.		;		mm Hg

Suspected abnormality: Normal

Comments:

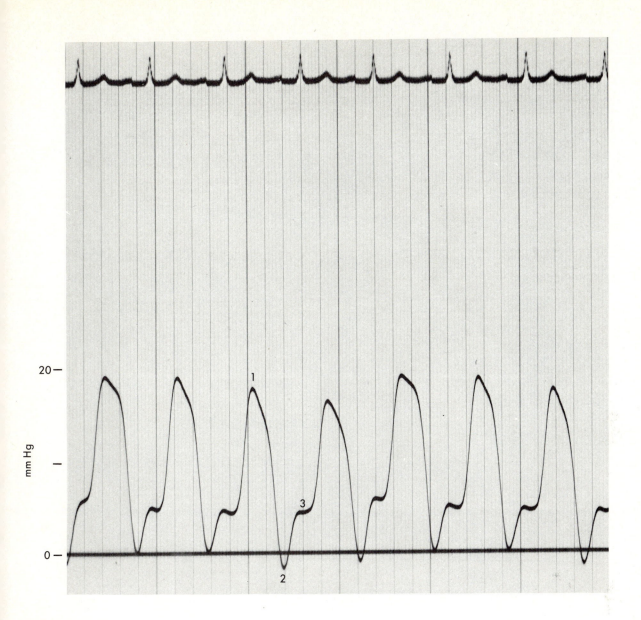

ANALYSIS

Rhythm: NSR

Pressure(s): RV

Waveform characteristics and measurements:

1.	RV systolic	;	18 mm Hg
2.	RV diastolic dip	;	0 mm Hg
3.	RV end-diastolic	;	5 mm Hg
4.		;	mm Hg
5.		;	mm Hg
6.		;	mm Hg
7.		;	mm Hg

Suspected abnormality: Normal

Comments:

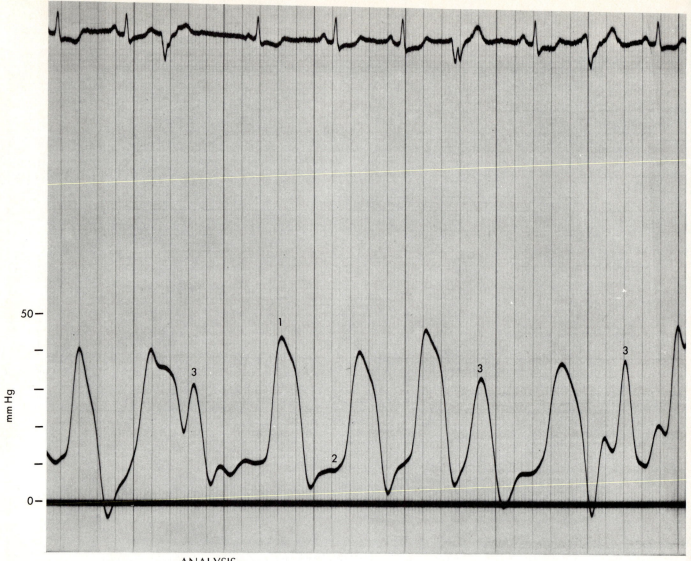

ANALYSIS

Rhythm: NSR with PVCs

Pressure(s): RV

Waveform characteristics and measurements:

1.	RV systolic	;	40	mm Hg
2.	RV end-diastolic	;	11	mm Hg
3.	PVC	;		mm Hg
4.		;		mm Hg
5.		;		mm Hg
6.		;		mm Hg
7.		;		mm Hg

Suspected abnormality: Right-sided heart failure

Comments: Note the effect of PVCs on the pressure contour of the RV. The elevated end-diastolic pressure of 11 mm Hg indicates RV failure; the elevated systolic pressure of 40 mm Hg suggests that the failure may be due to an increase in resistance to ejection either from pulmonary disease, mitral valve disease, or left-sided heart failure.

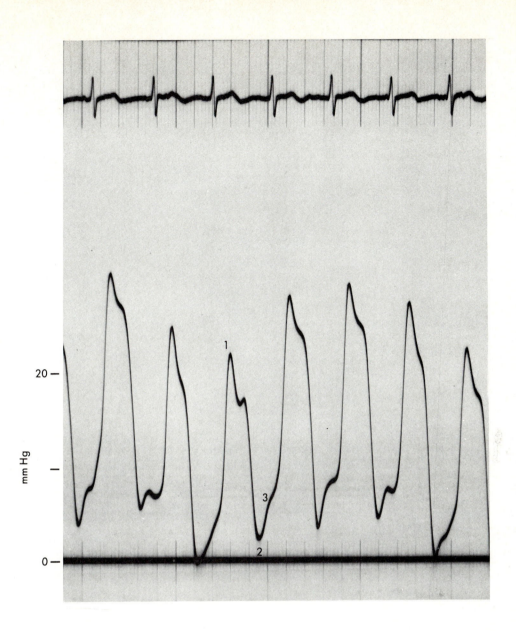

ANALYSIS

Rhythm: Regular supraventricular tachycardia

Pressure(s): RV

Waveform characteristics and measurements:

1.	RV systolic	; 26	mm Hg
2.	RV diastolic dip	; 2	mm Hg
3.	RV end-diastolic	; 6	mm Hg
4.		;	mm Hg
5.		;	mm Hg
6.		;	mm Hg
7.		;	mm Hg

Suspected abnormality: Normal

Comments:

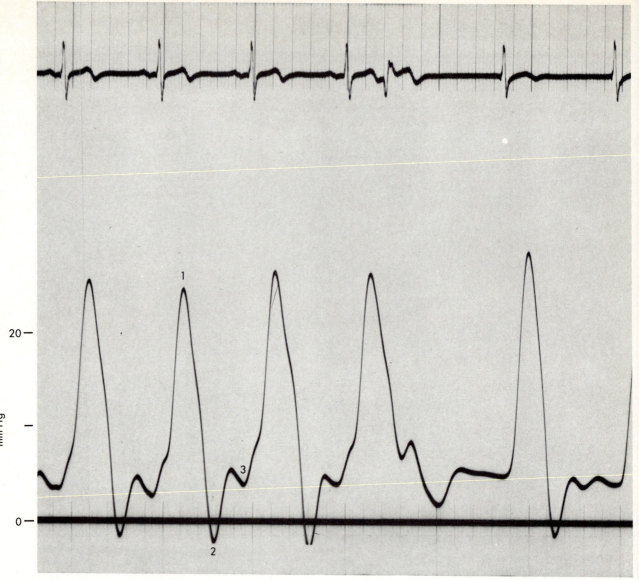

ANALYSIS

Rhythm: NSR with premature beat

Pressure(s): RV

Waveform characteristics and measurements:

1.	RV systolic	;	26 mm Hg
2.	RV early diastole	;	mm Hg
3.	RV end-diastolic	;	5 mm Hg
4.		;	mm Hg
5.		;	mm Hg
6.		;	mm Hg
7.		;	mm Hg

Suspected abnormality: Normal

Comments: Note the slightly higher RV systolic pressure in the next sinus beat after the premature beat. This is due to prolonged diastolic filling time as a result of the increased RR interval.

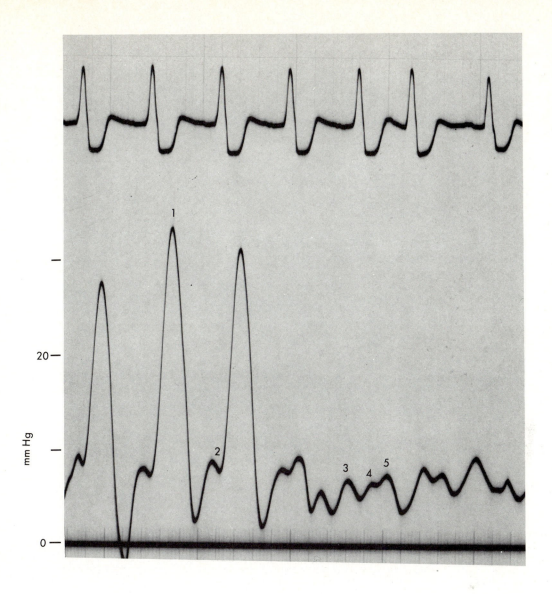

ANALYSIS

Rhythm: NSR with APC

Pressure(s): RV to RA

Waveform characteristics and measurements:

1.	RV systolic	;	30	mm Hg
2.	RV end-diastolic	;	8	mm Hg
3.	RA *a* wave	;	8	mm Hg
4.	RA *c* wave	;		mm Hg
5.	RA *v* wave	;	8	mm Hg
6.	RA mean	;	6	mm Hg
7.		;		mm Hg

Suspected abnormality: Mild RV failure

Comments:

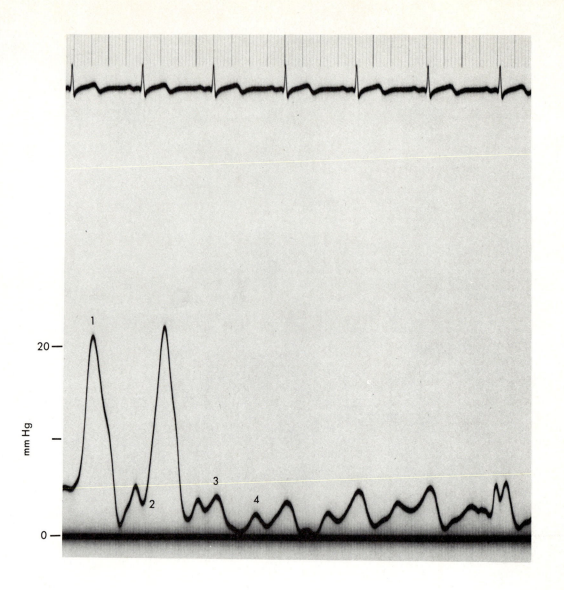

ANALYSIS

Rhythm: NSR

Pressure(s): RV to RA

Waveform characteristics and measurements:

1.	RV systolic	;	22	mm Hg
2.	RV end-diastolic	;	3	mm Hg
3.	RA *a* wave	;	3	mm Hg
4.	RA *v* wave	;	2	mm Hg
5.	RA mean	;	3	mm Hg
6.		;		mm Hg
7.		;		mm Hg

Suspected abnormality: Normal

Comments:

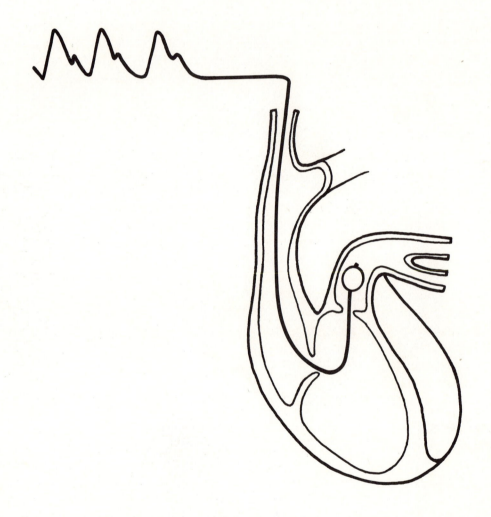

chapter 3

Pulmonary artery pressures

Physiology and morphology

The pulmonary artery (PA) pressure is divided into two phases: systole and diastole. Systole begins with the opening of the pulmonic valve, resulting in rapid ejection of blood into the pulmonary artery. On the PA pressure tracing this is seen as a sharp rise in pressure, followed by a decline in pressure as the volume decreases. When the RV pressure falls below the level of the PA pressure, the pulmonic valve snaps shut. This sudden closure of the valve leaflets produces a small rise on the downslope of the PA pressure and is termed the *dicrotic notch*. The systolic value referred to is the peak systolic pressure reached. Normal PA systolic pressure is 20 to 30 mm Hg.

Diastole follows closure of the pulmonic valve. During this time, runoff to the pulmonary system occurs without any further blood flow from the right ventricle until the next systole. The PA diastolic value referred to is the end-diastolic pressure just prior to the next systole. This value corresponds closely to the LV end-diastolic pressure (LVedp) in the absence of pulmonary disease or mitral valve disease. Normal PA end-diastolic pressure is 8 to 12 mm Hg.

ECG correlation

The systolic phase of the PA pressure should correspond closely to ventricular depolarization. However, catheter length and the amount of tubing used can delay this considerably. Generally, it occurs in the QT interval of the ECG.

In atrial fibrillation the value of the PA pressure varies greatly (p. 44), depending on the RR intervals and length of time for ventricular filling. The shorter the RR interval, the shorter the ventricular filling time, the less stroke volume ejected, and the less pressure rise in the PA. The contour of the PA pressure tracing remains normal, however.

Abnormal findings

Certain pathologic conditions alter the PA pressure. Pulmonary disease or essential pulmonary hypertension elevates the PA pressure due to an increase in pulmonary vascular resistance. Mitral valve disease and LV failure increase pulmonary venous pressure which in turn increases the PA pressure. Intracardiac left-to-right shunts, either atrial or ventricular, increase pulmonary blood flow and PA pressure. Hypoxia increases pulmonary vascular resistance and therefore PA pressure.

In general, the PAedp correlates closely with the PAW pressure. This allows us to more safely monitor the PAedp as a reflection of LVedp and avoid obtaining repeated PAW pressures with its inherent risks of damage to the pulmonary vasculature, including hemorrhage, ischemia, and pulmonary infarction. There are some situations, however, in which there is a wide discrepancy between the PAedp and PAW pressures. As mentioned previously, pulmonary disease elevates pulmonary artery pressure but usually does not affect the PAW pressure, which is a reflection of LA pressure, i.e., distal to the level of increased resistance. Pulmonary embolus also increases resistance and therefore increases PA pressure without affecting the PAW pressure. Very rapid heart rates elevate the PA diastolic pressure by abbreviating the duration of the diastolic period. In all these situations it may be necessary to use the PAW pressure to monitor LVedp.

In addition to pathologic abnormalities, mechanical abnormalities frequently alter the PA pressure both in contour and value. "Fling" or "whip" in the PA pressure tracing (p. 41), consisting of exaggerated oscillations, can occur with excessive catheter coiling in either the RA or RV or when the catheter tip is located near the pulmonic valve, where blood flow is turbulent. Patients with pulmonary hypertension and dilated pulmonary arteries frequently exhibit fling in the PA pressure tracing. In these situations accurate measurement of the PA pressure is difficult, and manipulation and repositioning of the catheter are necessary.

Damping of the PA pressure, due to a variety of causes, changes both the contour and the value of the PA waveform in a characteristic manner. The entire waveform loses any sharp definition and becomes rather rounded out in appearance. Frequently the upstroke of the systolic pressure is slow and the dicrotic notch is absent or poorly defined. The value of the PA pressure is decreased considerably and as such is an inaccurate pressure. Most often fibrin at the tip of the catheter is the culprit when pressures become damped. Careful aspiration followed by gentle flushing usually corrects this problem, but occasionally catheter replacement is necessary. Placement of the tip of the catheter against the wall of the vessel also produces damped pressures and requires repositioning of the catheter. The presence of an air bubble(s) anywhere within the system also dampens the pressure waveform. Kinks in either the catheter itself or the extension tubing produce a dampened, lowered pressure waveform.

The use of positive pressure mechanical ventilation artifactually increases the PA pressure. Measurement of the PA pressure both on and off the ventilator reveals the pressure alterations caused by ventilator assistance in addition to the actual PA pressure. Frequently this maneuver results in severe hypoxemia. Trend monitoring of the PA pressure is still possible and useful.

Examples

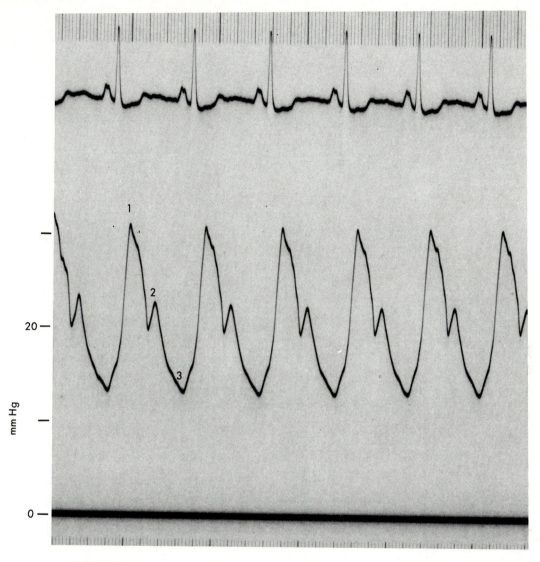

ANALYSIS

Rhythm: NSR

Pressure(s): PA

Waveform characteristics and measurements:

1.	PA systolic	;	30 mm Hg
2.	Dicrotic notch	;	mm Hg
3.	PA end-diastolic	;	13 mm Hg
4.		;	mm Hg
5.		;	mm Hg
6.		;	mm Hg
7.		;	mm Hg

Suspected abnormality: Normal

Comments:

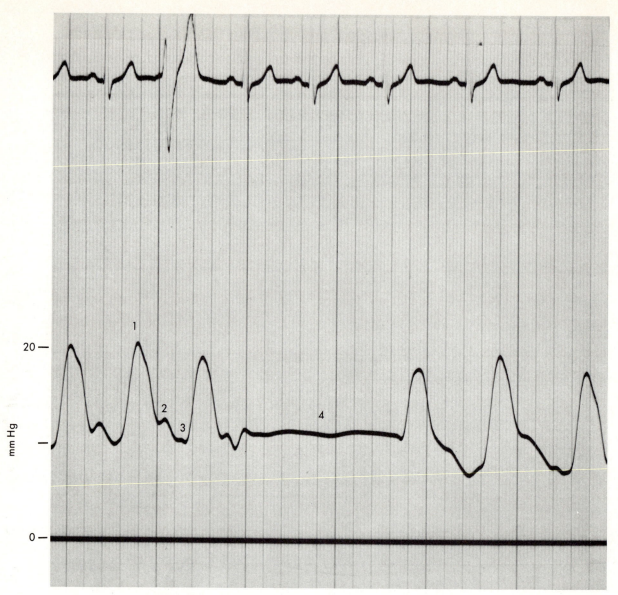

ANALYSIS

Rhythm: NSR with PVC

Pressure(s): PA

Waveform characteristics and measurements:

#	Characteristic		Value	
1.	PA systolic	;	20	mm Hg
2.	Dicrotic notch	;		mm Hg
3.	PA end-diastolic	;	9	mm Hg
4.	PA mean	;	12	mm Hg
5.		;		mm Hg
6.		;		mm Hg
7.		;		mm Hg

Suspected abnormality: Normal

Comments: Because diastole comprises approximately two thirds of the cardiac cycle, the average or mean of the PA pressure is much closer to the diastolic value than the systolic value.

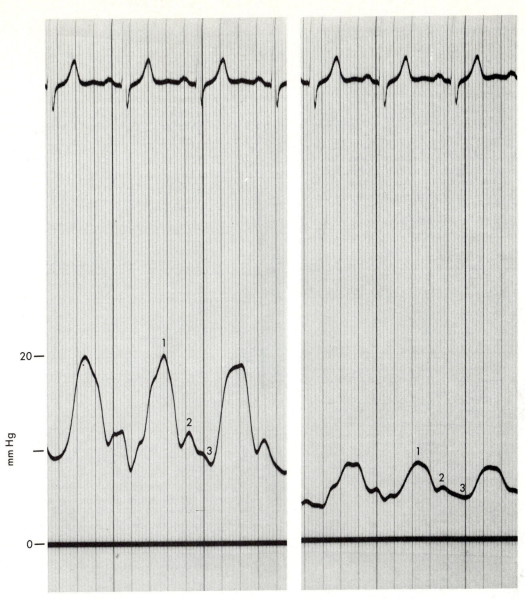

ANALYSIS

Rhythm: NSR

Pressure(s): PA

Waveform characteristics and measurements:

1.	PA systolic ;	20 (8) mm Hg
2.	Dicrotic notch ;	mm Hg
3.	PA end-diastolic ;	9 (4) mm Hg
4.	;	mm Hg
5.	;	mm Hg
6.	;	mm Hg
7.	;	mm Hg

Suspected abnormality: Normal and damped

Comments: Note the damping effect in the latter three pressure waveforms due to a clot at the tip of the catheter or an air bubble within the system. Note the similar contour of the pressure tracings, with a marked decrease in value.

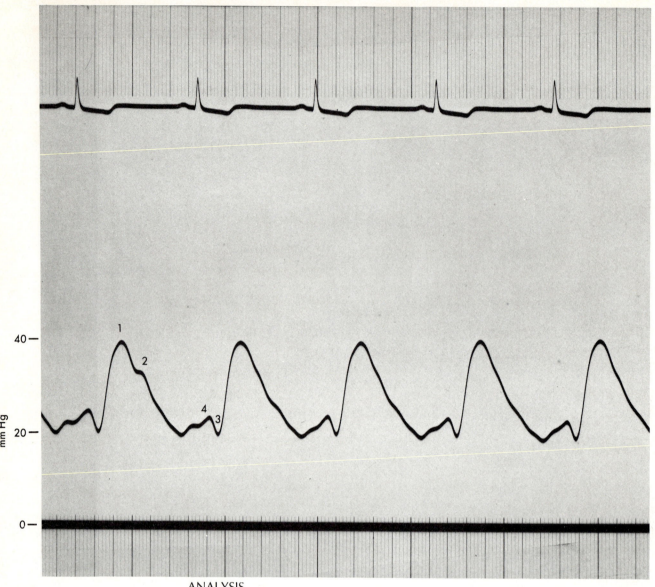

ANALYSIS

Rhythm: NSR

Pressure(s): PA

Waveform characteristics and measurements:

1.	PA systolic	;	40	mm Hg
2.	Dicrotic notch	;		mm Hg
3.	*a* Wave reflected back from LA	;		mm Hg
4.	PA end-diastolic	;	20	mm Hg
5.		;		mm Hg
6.		;		mm Hg
7.		;		mm Hg

Suspected abnormality: Mild CHF

Comments: This PA pressure waveform is somewhat damped with a rounded-out appearance and poorly defined dicrotic notch. It is possible, at times, to see retrograde transmission of the LA *a* wave.

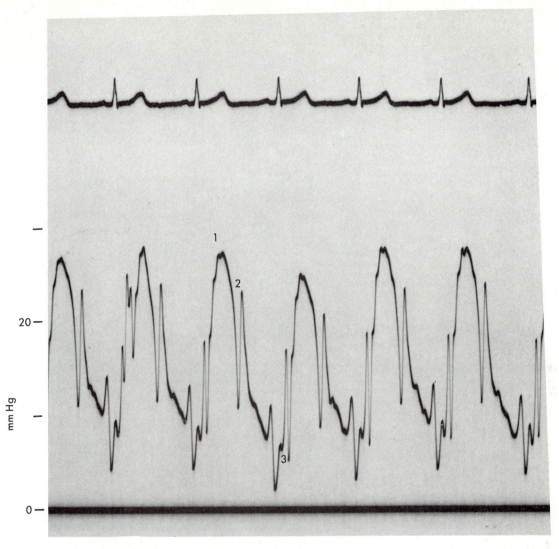

ANALYSIS

Rhythm: NSR

Pressure(s): PA

Waveform characteristics and measurements:

1.	PA systolic	;	26	mm Hg
2.	Dicrotic notch	;		mm Hg
3.	PA end-diastolic	;	(?) 9	mm Hg
4.		;		mm Hg
5.		;		mm Hg
6.		;		mm Hg
7.		;		mm Hg

Suspected abnormality: Normal

Comments: This PA pressure is of normal value with abnormal contour due to catheter "fling," making accurate identification of PA end-diastolic pressure difficult.

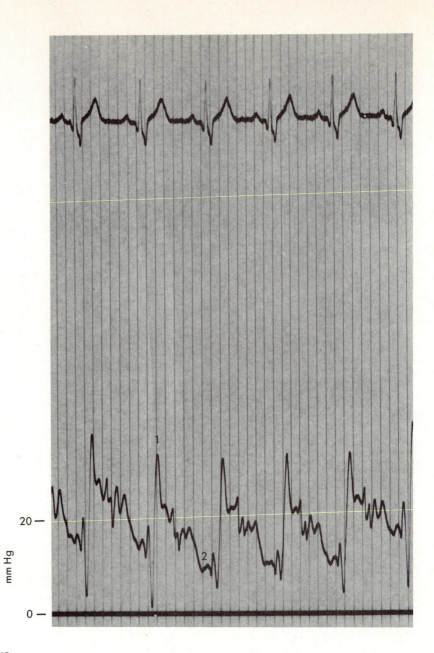

ANALYSIS

Rhythm: NSR

Pressure(s): PA

Waveform characteristics and measurements:

1.	PA systolic	;	30	mm Hg
2.	PA end-diastolic	;	(?) 10	mm Hg
3.		;		mm Hg
4.		;		mm Hg
5.		;		mm Hg
6.		;		mm Hg
7.		;		mm Hg

Suspected abnormality: Normal

Comments: Note the "fling" or "noise" in this PA waveform, producing many small oscillations, in addition to a sharp negative wave occurring just prior to the systolic upstroke. This is due to catheter fling and can be misinterpreted as the PAedp by the monitoring system.

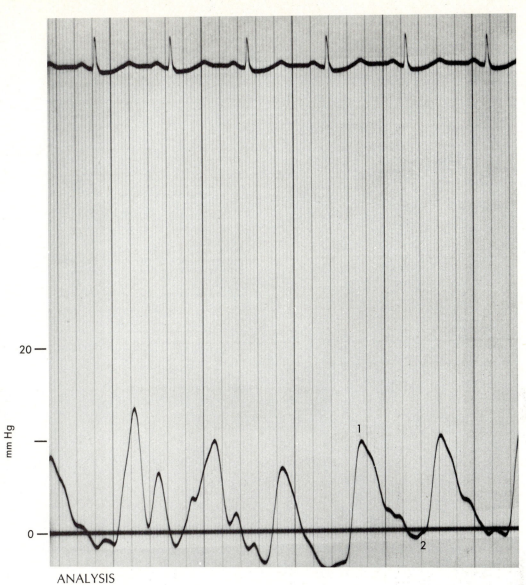

ANALYSIS

Rhythm: NSR

Pressure(s): PA

Waveform characteristics and measurements:

1.	PA systolic	;	10 mm Hg
2.	PA diastolic	;	0 mm Hg
3.		;	mm Hg
4.		;	mm Hg
5.		;	mm Hg
6.		;	mm Hg
7.		;	mm Hg

Suspected abnormality: Artifactual pressure

Comments: This artifactually low pressure is due to incorrect placement of the transducer above the level of the right atrium. Because the diastolic pressure falls to or even below the baseline (zero), this PA pressure tracing could be confused with an RV pressure tracing. However, closer scrutiny reveals a normal PA contour with systole, dicrotic notch, and runoff in diastole.

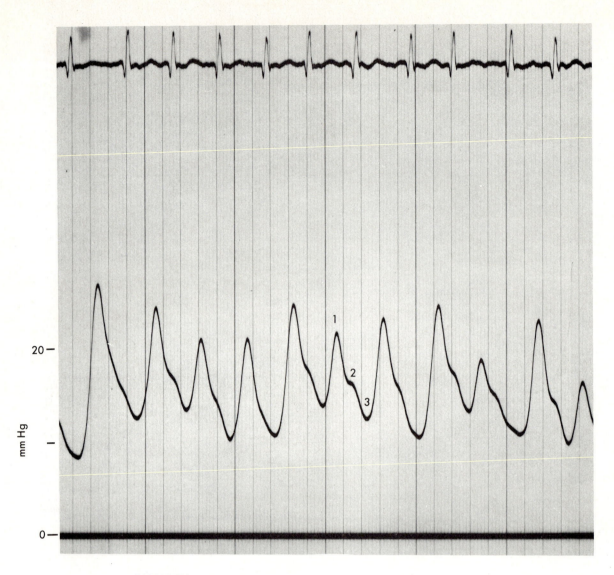

ANALYSIS

Rhythm: Atrial fibrillation

Pressure(s): PA

Waveform characteristics and measurements:

1.	PA systolic	;	19-24	mm Hg
2.	Dicrotic notch	;		mm Hg
3.	PA end-diastolic	;	9-14	mm Hg
4.		;		mm Hg
5.		;		mm Hg
6.		;		mm Hg
7.		;		mm Hg

Suspected abnormality: Normal

Comments: Note varying PA systolic pressure secondary to varying RR intervals and length of time for diastolic filling to occur.

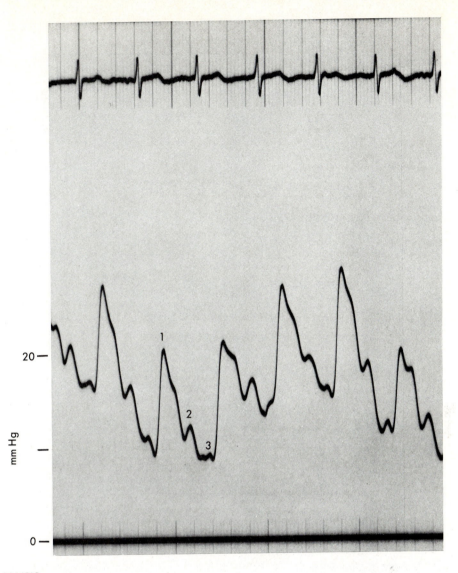

ANALYSIS

Rhythm: Regular supraventricular tachycardia

Pressure(s): PA

Waveform characteristics and measurements:

1.	PA systolic	;	25 mm Hg
2.	Dicrotic notch	;	mm Hg
3.	PA end-diastolic	;	12 mm Hg
4.		;	mm Hg
5.		;	mm Hg
6.		;	mm Hg
7.		;	mm Hg

Suspected abnormality: Normal

Comments: Note the exaggerated, but normal, respiratory variation in this PA pressure tracing, with the end-diastolic value ranging from a low of 9 mm Hg to a high of 15 mm Hg. A more accurate reading can be obtained by asking the patient to quietly suspend respirations at the very end of expiration and record the PA pressure at that time. Since this is not usually feasible, it is possible to average the values over at least two respiratory cycles, as done in this case, or record the pressure at end-expiration.

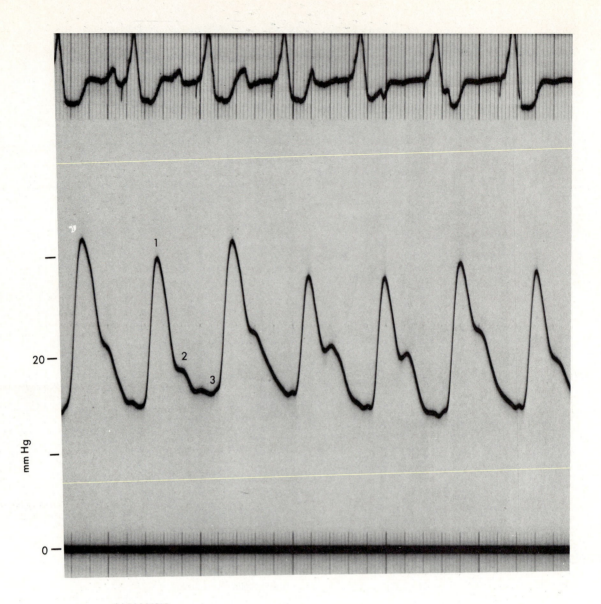

ANALYSIS

Rhythm: Paced (Note pacemaker spikes and P waves throughout ECG.)

Pressure(s): PA

Waveform characteristics and measurements:

1.	PA systolic	;	31		mm Hg
2.	Dicrotic notch	;			mm Hg
3.	PA end-diastolic	;	16		mm Hg
4.		;			mm Hg
5.		;			mm Hg
6.		;			mm Hg
7.		;			mm Hg

Suspected abnormality: Mild CHF

Comments:

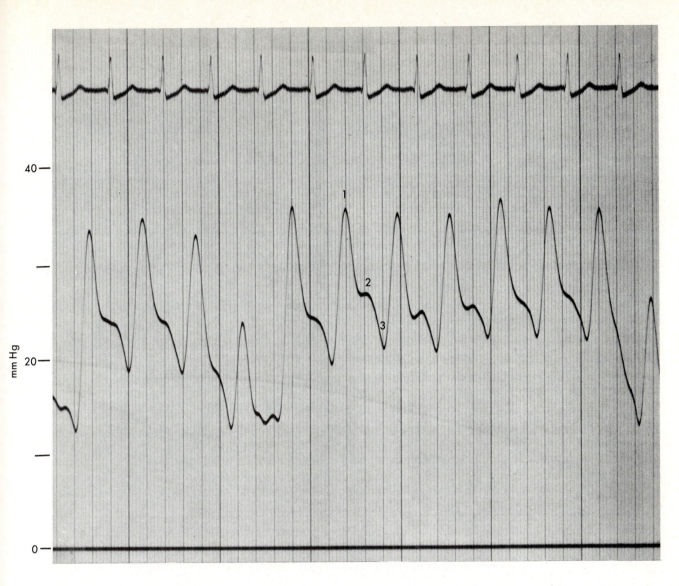

ANALYSIS

Rhythm: NSR

Pressure(s): PA

Waveform characteristics and measurements:

1.	PA systolic	;	35	mm Hg
2.	Dicrotic notch	;		mm Hg
3.	PA end-diastolic	;	20	mm Hg
4.		;		mm Hg
5.		;		mm Hg
6.		;		mm Hg
7.		;		mm Hg

Suspected abnormality: Pulmonary disease

Comments: The mildly elevated PA pressure of 35/20 is due to increased PVR occurring in pulmonary disease. This pressure does not reflect left-sided heart pressures. Therefore the PAW pressure, instead of the PAedp, should be monitored to reflect LVedp. Note the marked drop in PA pressure during inspiration.

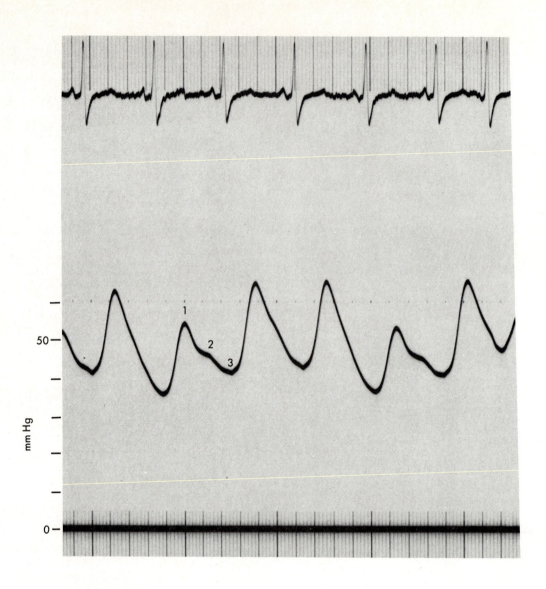

ANALYSIS

Rhythm: NSR

Pressure(s): PA

Waveform characteristics and measurements:

1.	PA systolic	;	60	mm Hg
2.	Dicrotic notch	;		mm Hg
3.	PA end-diastolic	;	40	mm Hg
4.		;		mm Hg
5.		;		mm Hg
6.		;		mm Hg
7.		;		mm Hg

Suspected abnormality: Pulmonary hypertension

Comments: This PA waveform appears damped, a frequent finding in patients with this disease and high PVR. Note pressure changes due to respiratory variation.

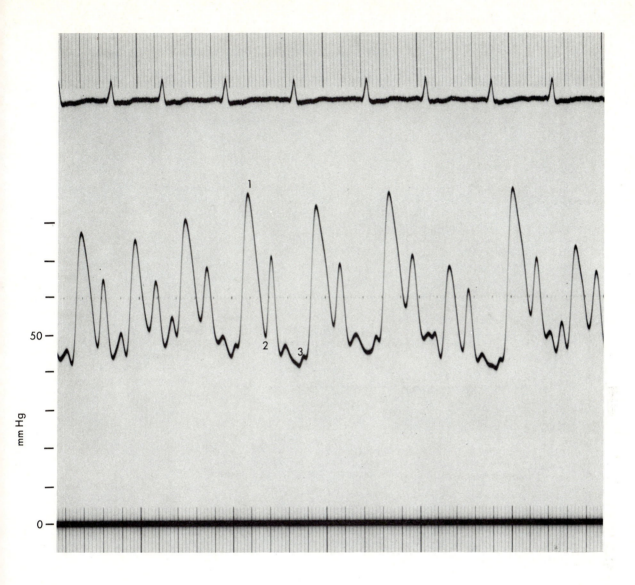

ANALYSIS

Rhythm: Atrial fibrillation

Pressure(s): PA

Waveform characteristics and measurements:

1.	PA systolic	; 80	mm Hg
2.	Dicrotic notch	;	mm Hg
3.	PA end-diastolic	; 42	mm Hg
4.		;	mm Hg
5.		;	mm Hg
6.		;	mm Hg
7.		;	mm Hg

Suspected abnormality: Pulmonary hypertension secondary to severe COPD

Comments: Note exaggerated pressure changes due to noncompliant pulmonary vasculature with pulmonary hypertension.

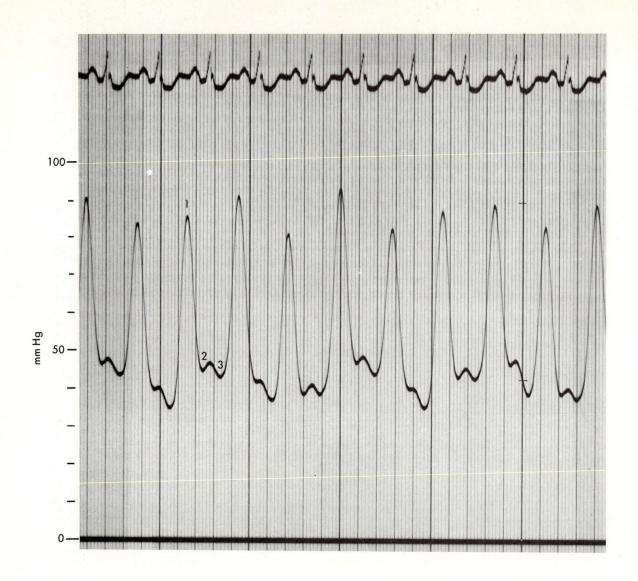

ANALYSIS

Rhythm: Sinus tachycardia

Pressure(s): PA

Waveform characteristics and measurements:

1.	PA systolic	;	87 mm Hg
2.	Dicrotic notch	;	mm Hg
3.	PA end-diastolic	;	40 mm Hg
4.		;	mm Hg
5.		;	mm Hg
6.		;	mm Hg
7.		;	mm Hg

Suspected abnormality: Pulmonary hypertension secondary to severe mitral stenosis and mitral regurgitation

Comments: Note the abbreviated diastolic phase due to the tachycardia.

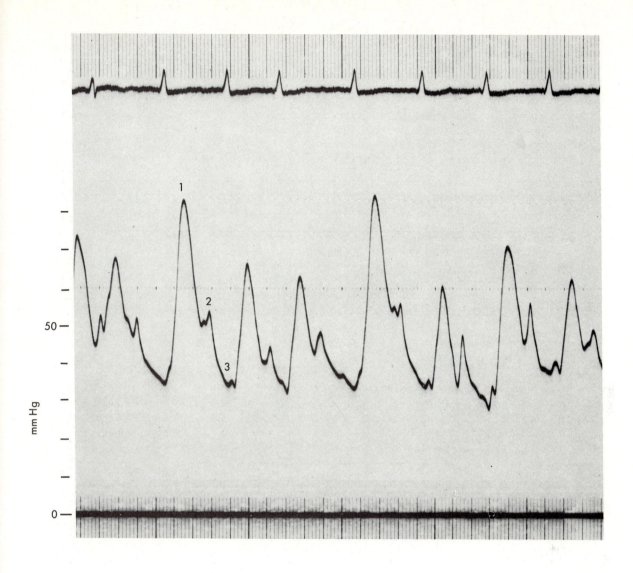

ANALYSIS

Rhythm: Atrial fibrillation

Pressure(s): PA

Waveform characteristics and measurements:

1.	PA systolic	; 72	mm Hg
2.	Dicrotic notch	;	mm Hg
3.	PA end-diastolic	; 32	mm Hg
4.		;	mm Hg
5.		;	mm Hg
6.		;	mm Hg
7.		;	mm Hg

Suspected abnormality: Severe pulmonary hypertension secondary to mitral regurgitation and CHF

Comments:

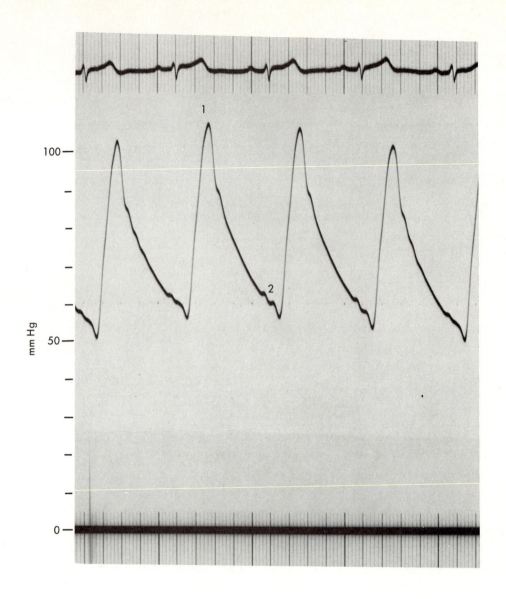

ANALYSIS

Rhythm: NSR

Pressure(s): PA

Waveform characteristics and measurements:

1.	PA systolic	;	105 mm Hg
2.	PA end-diastolic	;	55 mm Hg
3.		;	mm Hg
4.		;	mm Hg
5.		;	mm Hg
6.		;	mm Hg
7.		;	mm Hg

Suspected abnormality: Severe pulmonary hypertension

Comments:

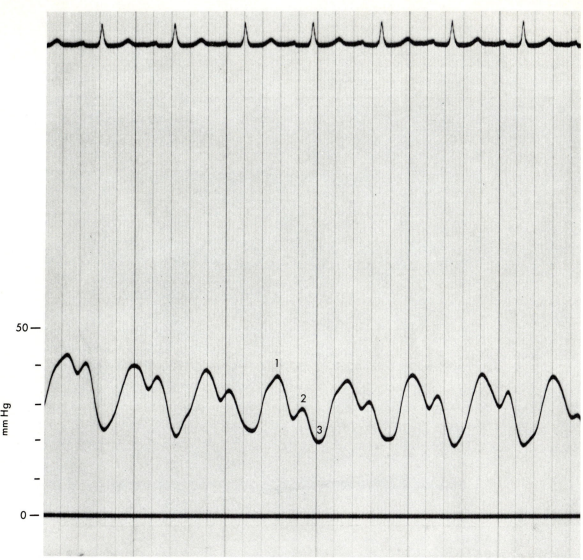

ANALYSIS

Rhythm: NSR

Pressure(s): PA

Waveform characteristics and measurements:

1.	PA systolic	;	40	mm Hg
2.	(?) *v* Wave reflected from LA	;		mm Hg
3.	PA end-diastolic	;	20	mm Hg
4.		;		mm Hg
5.		;		mm Hg
6.		;		mm Hg
7.		;		mm Hg

Suspected abnormality: CHF, (?) mitral regurgitation

Comments: This PA pressure has an unusual contour that may be due to a superimposed *v* wave reflected back from the LA. Evaluation of the PAW pressure contour and value is necessary to confirm this.

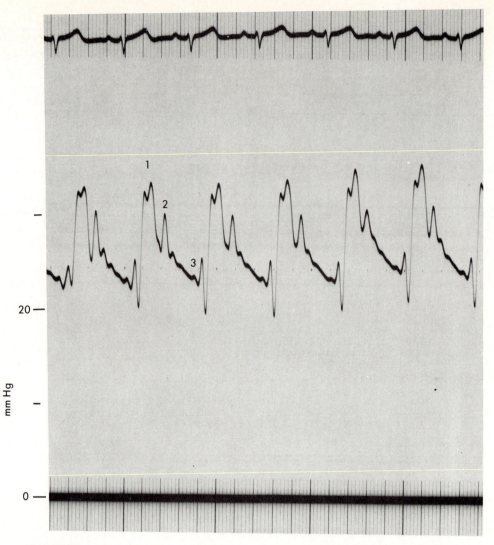

ANALYSIS

Rhythm: NSR

Pressure(s): PA

Waveform characteristics and measurements:

1.	PA systolic	;	34	mm Hg
2.	Dicrotic notch	;		mm Hg
3.	PA end-diastolic	;	22	mm Hg
4.		;		mm Hg
5.		;		mm Hg
6.		;		mm Hg
7.		;		mm Hg

Suspected abnormality: LV failure

Comments: Nitroprusside therapy has markedly reduced this patient's pulmonary hypertension, but the vasodilation and increased turbulent flow produce much noise or fling in the pressure contour. Advancing the catheter a bit further sometimes remedies this problem. The noise or fling in this case makes it difficult to accurately identify the PA end-diastolic pressure.

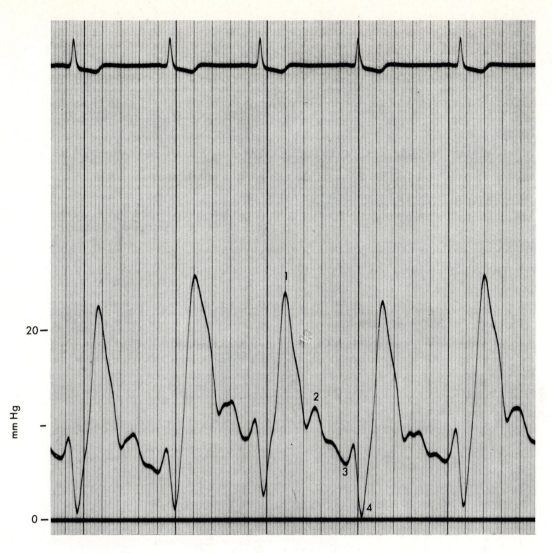

ANALYSIS

Rhythm: Atrial fibrillation

Pressure(s): PA/RV

Waveform characteristics and measurements:

1.	PA systolic	;	24	mm Hg
2.	Dicrotic notch	;		mm Hg
3.	PA end-diastolic	;	9	mm Hg
4.	RV diastolic	;	1	mm Hg
5.		;		mm Hg
6.		;		mm Hg
7.		;		mm Hg

Suspected abnormality: Normal

Comments: The countour of this pressure waveform has the appearance of a mixed PA/RV pressure with the diastolic pressure coming down to baseline. This is due to location of the catheter tip right at the pulmonic valve, which results in forward movement of the catheter into the PA during systole and backward movement of the catheter into the RV during diastole. Inflation of the balloon of the catheter should allow the catheter to float out to the PA.

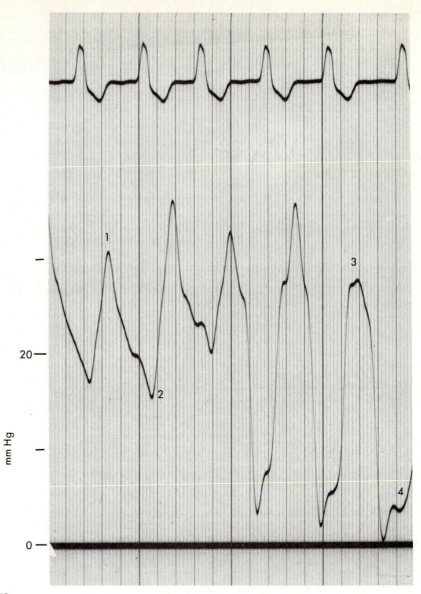

ANALYSIS

Rhythm: Atrial fibrillation

Pressure(s): PA to RV

Waveform characteristics and measurements:

1.	PA systolic	;	32 mm Hg
2.	PA end-diastolic	;	18 mm Hg
3.	RV systolic	;	30 mm Hg
4.	RV end-diastolic	;	6 mm Hg
5.		;	mm Hg
6.		;	mm Hg
7.		;	mm Hg

Suspected abnormality: Normal

Comments: The catheter has slipped from the PA back into the RV. Inflation of the balloon should carry the tip of the catheter back into the PA. If this does not occur, the catheter must be withdrawn out of the RV. Note the normal respiratory variation in both pressures.

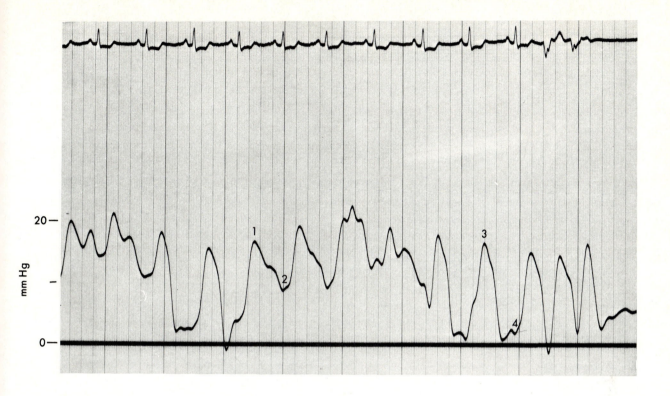

ANALYSIS

Rhythm: NSR with PVCs

Pressure(s): PA and RV

Waveform characteristics and measurements:

1.	PA systolic	;	19	mm Hg
2.	PA end-diastolic	;	10	mm Hg
3.	RV systolic	;	17	mm Hg
4.	RV end-diastolic	;	2	mm Hg
5.		;		mm Hg
6.		;		mm Hg
7.		;		mm Hg

Suspected abnormality: Normal

Comments: The tip of the catheter is located at the pulmonic valve, moving back and forth across the valve and producing PA and RV pressure waveforms. It is not in a safe location for monitoring purposes (note the occurrence of PVCs). It would also be impossible to obtain a PAW pressure waveform with the catheter tip in this location. Frequently inflation of the balloon will carry the catheter tip out distally to the PA. Unfortunately it is usually not carried distally enough to obtain a PAW pressure, but safe monitoring of the PA pressure can be continued.

57

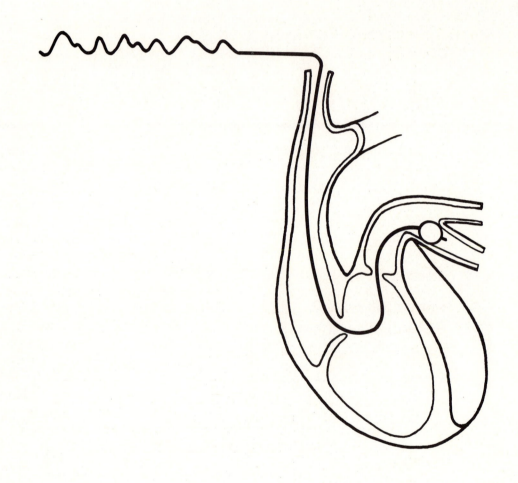

chapter 4

Pulmonary artery wedge pressures

Physiology and morphology

When proper position in a small branch of the PA is achieved, inflation of the balloon of the Swan-Ganz catheter actually occludes flow and therefore pressure in that segment of the pulmonary artery. The pressure obtained with balloon inflation is termed the *pulmonary artery wedge (PAW)*. This pressure reflects left atrial (LA) pressure and has similar contour and characteristics as the right atrial pressure, since the pressure is produced by the same physiologic events. The *a* wave of the PAW pressure is produced by LA systole and is followed by the *x* descent, reflecting a decrease in left atrial volume following systole. The *c* wave that is produced by closure of the mitral valve frequently gets lost in retrograde transmission and often is not observed in the PAW pressure waveform. The *v* wave is produced by filling of the LA and bulging back of the mitral valve during ventricular systole. The decline succeeding the *v* wave is the *y* descent, which represents opening of the mitral valve with a decrease in LA pressure and volume during passive emptying into the LV.

Although the contour of the PAW pressure is the same as the RA pressure, the value of the PAW pressure is normally higher. As with the RA pressure, we generally record the mean of the PAW pressure, since the *a* and *v* waves are normally of approximately the same value. The normal resting PAW mean pressure is 4 to 12 mm Hg. If, however, either the *a* or the *v* wave is particularly dominant or elevated, it is not accurate to average the pressure rises. In those instances the value of both the *a* wave and the *v* wave should be noted.

ECG correlation

Timing of the electrical and mechanical events is the same as with the RA pressure, i.e., the *a* wave follows the P wave of the ECG, and the *v* wave follows the T wave of the ECG. However, a greater time delay between electrical and mechanical events is frequently noted with the PAW pressure.

The effects of arrhythmias on the PAW pressure are the same as those discussed with the RA pressure. In atrial fibrillation there are no *a* waves in the

PAW pressure waveform, and only a *v* wave follows each QRS complex. Junctional rhythm or AV dissociation can produce giant or cannon *a* waves.

Abnormal findings

Elevated PAW pressures occur in the following conditions:
1. LV failure
2. Mitral stenosis or regurgitation
3. Cardiac tamponade
4. Constrictive pericarditis
5. Volume overload

The *a* wave of the PAW pressure is exaggerated and elevated in any condition that increases the resistance to LV filling. Elevation of the PAW *a* wave with LV failure reflects the increased filling pressure required with elevated LV diastolic pressures. In pure mitral stenosis the PAW *a* wave is dominant and elevated due to the resistance met at the narrowed mitral orifice. It represents the increased force of contraction required to eject blood through the stenotic valve. The *y* descent of the PAW pressure is usually prolonged in mitral stenosis, indicating increased resistance to passive filling of the LV.

The *v* wave of the PAW pressure is exaggerated and elevated with mitral insufficiency due to regurgitation of blood back into the LA during ventricular systole. Mitral regurgitation can occur in varying degrees of severity and from a variety of causes. A mildly elevated and dominant *v* wave is commonly seen with LV failure and dilatation. Rheumatic fever or bacterial endocarditis can cause destruction to the valve leaflets and produce mitral regurgitation. Acute mitral regurgitation, with giant *v* waves, can occur with ruptured papillary muscle following myocardial infarction. On a lesser scale, ischemia of the papillary muscle can occur resulting in mild to moderate mitral regurgitation and elevation of the *v* wave.

In cardiac tamponade, constrictive pericardial disease, and hypervolemia the PAW *a* and *v* waves are elevated. In cardiac tamponade the *x* descent is prominent, whereas in constrictive pericarditis either the *y* descent is prominent or the *x* and *y* descents are equal, giving an M pattern to the PAW pressure waveform.

Hypovolemia produces a low PAW pressure. In the normal heart, PAW pressures less than 4 or 5 mm Hg indicate hypovolemia, whereas in the compromised heart, hypovolemia may be present with higher PAW pressures.

Mechanical abnormalities of the PAW pressure produce changes in both the value and the contour of the PAW pressure waveform. *Overwedging,* which is caused by overinflation or eccentric inflation of the balloon of the catheter or an exceedingly distal location of the catheter tip, may produce an artifactually elevated, damped, and inaccurate PAW pressure. In addition, there is usually a linear increase or decrease in the pressure waveform. (It resembles a line at an approximately 10- to 20-degree angle). Slow, careful, and accurate balloon inflation or, if the catheter is too distally positioned, withdrawal to a more proximal PA location may alleviate this problem.

Damping of the PAW pressure produces the same type of rounded-out appearance as with the PA pressure with lack of defined *a* or *v* waves. The balloon should be deflated before the catheter is aspirated and then gently flushed. Never flush in the PAW position.

Marked respiratory variation is often present in PAW pressure waveforms, making accurate interpretation somewhat difficult. This problem can be reduced by recording the PAW pressure at the end of the expiratory phase. Taking an average or mean of the pressure changes over two or three respiratory cycles also gives a more accurate reading.

The use of positive pressure ventilation also increases the measured PAW pressure. Measuring the PAW pressure both on and off the ventilator provides a more complete picture of the cardiac effects of increased intrathoracic pressure in addition to the actual, indirect ventricular filling pressure and volume. When this is not feasible, trend monitoring of the PAW pressure is still useful.

Occasionally a mixed PA/PAW pressure is obtained due to incomplete wedging of the catheter tip. Frequently the changes are directly related to respirations, with a PA pressure observed during expiration and a PAW pressure observed during inspiration. In this circumstance, slight advancement of the catheter is necessary to obtain an accurate PAW pressure.

Frequently, direct left atrial (LA) pressures are measured via a small catheter placed in the LA at the time of open heart surgery. Since the PAW pressure is an indirect measurement of LA pressure, both the contour and the value of the LA pressure are the same as the PAW pressure. The LA *a* wave, produced by left atrial systole, is followed by the *x* descent, a decline in pressure due to reduced LA volume. The *c* wave is produced by closure of the mitral valve leaflets and may or may not be evident in the LA waveform. The *v* wave results from filling of the LA and bulging back of the mitral valve during ventricular systole. This is followed by the *y* descent, reflecting a decrease in LA volume during passive filling of the LV. The delay between electrical and mechanical events that one sees in the PAW pressure is less apparent with the direct LA pressure, i.e., the LA *a* wave more immediately follows the P wave of the ECG.

Normal values for the LA pressure are a mean pressure of 4 to 12 mm Hg.

Examples

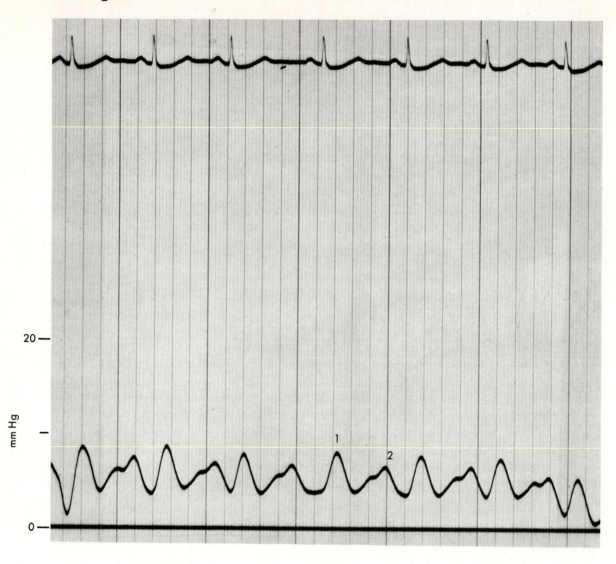

ANALYSIS

Rhythm: NSR

Pressure(s): PAW

Waveform characteristics and measurements:

1.	*a* Wave	;	8	mm Hg
2.	*v* Wave	;	7	mm Hg
3.	Mean	;	6	mm Hg
4.		;		mm Hg
5.		;		mm Hg
6.		;		mm Hg
7.		;		mm Hg

Suspected abnormality: Normal

Comments:

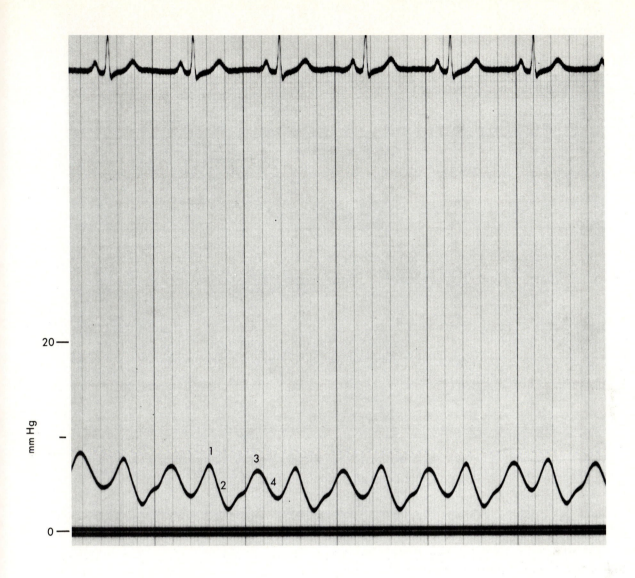

ANALYSIS

Rhythm: NSR

Pressure(s): PAW

Waveform characteristics and measurements:

1.	*a* Wave	;	8 mm Hg
2.	*x* Descent	;	mm Hg
3.	*v* Wave	;	8 mm Hg
4.	*y* Descent	;	mm Hg
5.	Mean	;	5 mm Hg
6.		;	mm Hg
7.		;	mm Hg

Suspected abnormality: Normal

Comments: Note the lack of respiratory variation seen when the patient momentarily suspends respirations at the end of expiration.

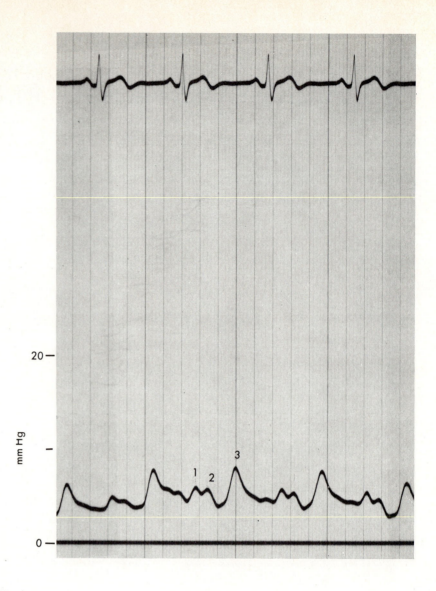

ANALYSIS

Rhythm: NSR

Pressure(s): PAW

Waveform characteristics and measurements:

1.	*a* Wave	;	5 mm Hg
2.	*c* Wave	;	mm Hg
3.	*v* Wave	;	8 mm Hg
4.	Mean	;	6 mm Hg
5.		;	mm Hg
6.		;	mm Hg
7.		;	mm Hg

Suspected abnormality: Normal or hypovolemia

Comments: This PAW pressure tracing falls within the normal range (mean of 6 mm Hg), albeit on the low side. If, however, this patient had evidence of a low cardiac output, this PAW pressure value would be considered too low, and this patient would warrant careful volume administration.

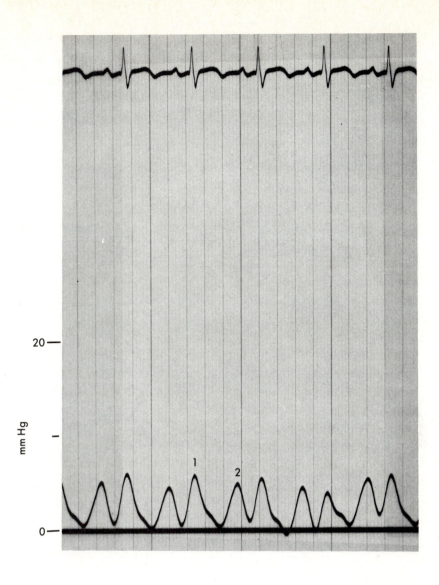

ANALYSIS

Rhythm: NSR

Pressure(s): PAW

Waveform characteristics and measurements:

1. _____ *a* Wave _____ ; _____ 5 _____ mm Hg

2. _____ *v* Wave _____ ; _____ 5 _____ mm Hg

3. _____ Mean _____ ; _____ 3 _____ mm Hg

4. _____ ; _____ mm Hg

5. _____ ; _____ mm Hg

6. _____ ; _____ mm Hg

7. _____ ; _____ mm Hg

Suspected abnormality: Hypovolemia

Comments: There is very little time delay between electrical and mechanical events (the *a* wave immediately succeeds the P wave). In this case a miniature transducer was connected directly to the catheter, eliminating all extension tubing.

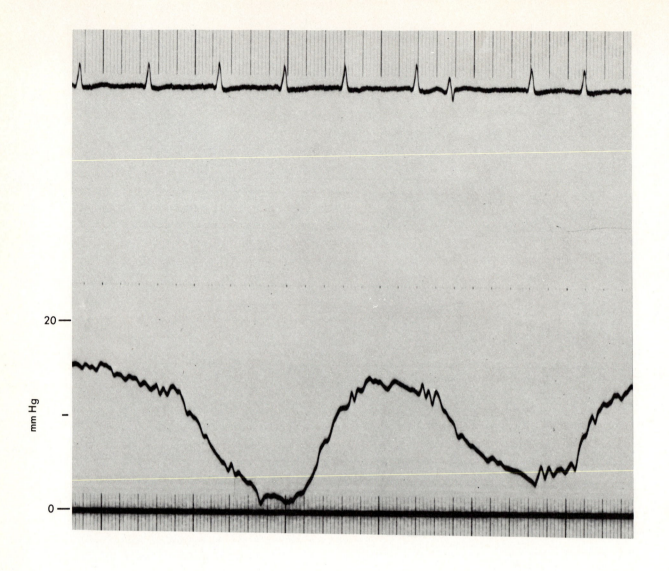

ANALYSIS

Rhythm: Atrial fibrillation

Pressure(s): PAW

Waveform characteristics and measurements:

1.	Mean	;	10 mm Hg
2.		;	mm Hg
3.		;	mm Hg
4.		;	mm Hg
5.		;	mm Hg
6.		;	mm Hg
7.		;	mm Hg

Suspected abnormality: Normal

Comments: This PAW is damped with marked respiratory variation, making accurate waveform identification difficult.

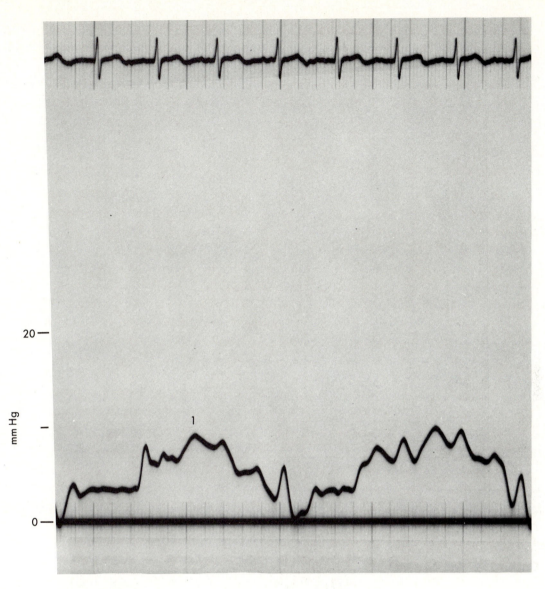

ANALYSIS

Rhythm: Regular supraventricular tachycardia

Pressure(s): PAW

Waveform characteristics and measurements:

1. _____ *v* Wave _____ ; _____ 6 _____ mm Hg
2. _____ Mean _____ ; _____ 6 _____ mm Hg
3. _____ ; _____ mm Hg
4. _____ ; _____ mm Hg
5. _____ ; _____ mm Hg
6. _____ ; _____ mm Hg
7. _____ ; _____ mm Hg

Suspected abnormality: Normal or hypovolemia

Comments: Note normal respiratory variation.

67

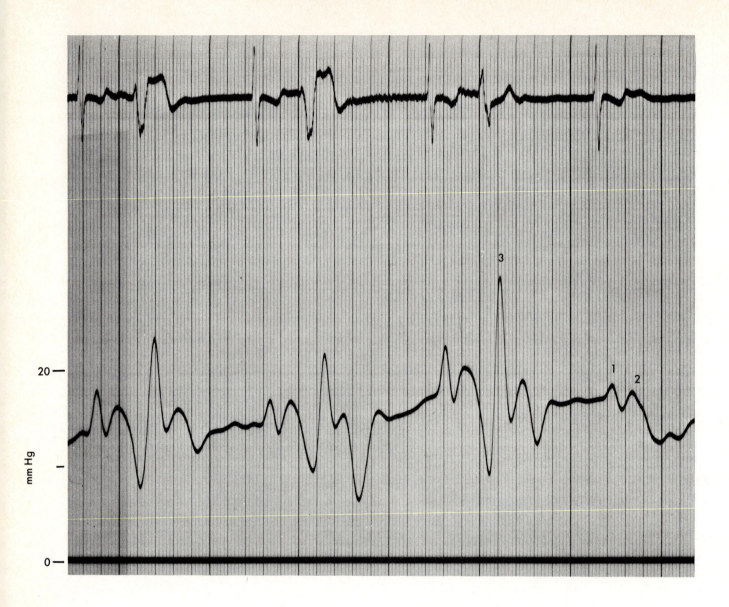

ANALYSIS

Rhythm: Supraventricular with PVCs

Pressure(s): PAW

Waveform characteristics and measurements:

1.	c Wave	;	_____ mm Hg
2.	v Wave	;	18 mm Hg
3.	v Wave 2° PVC	;	25-30 mm Hg
4.	Mean	;	16 mm Hg
5.	_____	;	_____ mm Hg
6.	_____	;	_____ mm Hg
7.	_____	;	_____ mm Hg

Suspected abnormality: Mild CHF

Comments: The prominent and elevated v wave following the premature ventricular contraction reflects an increase in LA volume when ventricular systole occurs while the mitral valve is open.

68

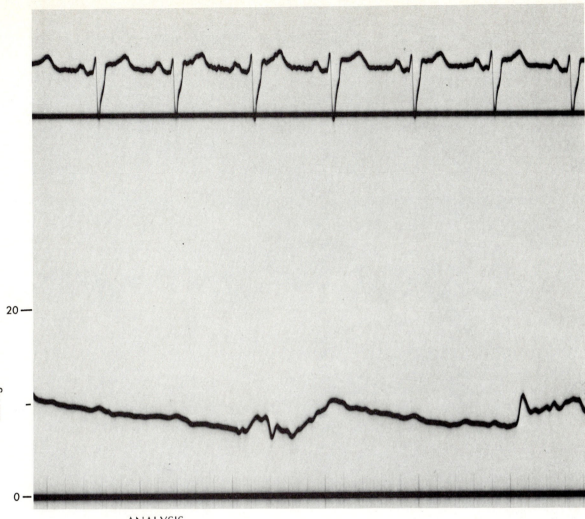

ANALYSIS

Rhythm: NSR

Pressure(s): (?) PAW

Waveform characteristics and measurements:

1. _____ ; _____ mm Hg

2. _____ ; _____ mm Hg

3. _____ ; _____ mm Hg

4. _____ ; _____ mm Hg

5. _____ ; _____ mm Hg

6. _____ ; _____ mm Hg

7. _____ ; _____ mm Hg

Suspected abnormality: Overwedged pressure

Comments: Overwedging occurs when the balloon of the catheter is inflated with an excessive amount of air for the size vessel in which the catheter is positioned. Characteristically, the pressure appears to angle either upward or downward, as in this case. Careful monitoring of the pressure waveforms during balloon inflation, with immediate cessation of inflation when a PAW waveform is obtained, can prevent this problem. If a PAW pressure waveform appears after inflation of only a small amount of air, the catheter may have advanced too far distally into a smaller caliber vessel and should be withdrawn slightly.

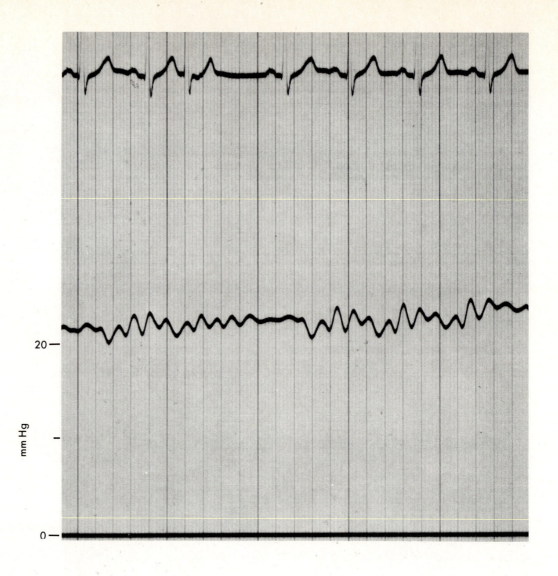

ANALYSIS

Rhythm: NSR with PNB

Pressure(s): PAW

Waveform characteristics and measurements:

1.	Mean	;	24 mm Hg
2.		;	mm Hg
3.		;	mm Hg
4.		;	mm Hg
5.		;	mm Hg
6.		;	mm Hg
7.		;	mm Hg

Suspected abnormality: Overinflation of the balloon

Comments: This damped PAW pressure tracing is the result of overinflation of the balloon of the Swan-Ganz catheter. Although the amount of air injected may not exceed the manufacturer's recommendation, it may exceed the size of the vessel the catheter tip lies in. When this occurs, the balloon itself can eccentrically inflate over the tip of the catheter, producing this damped, overwedged PAW pressure waveform. Careful observation of the waveform during balloon inflation can eliminate this problem.

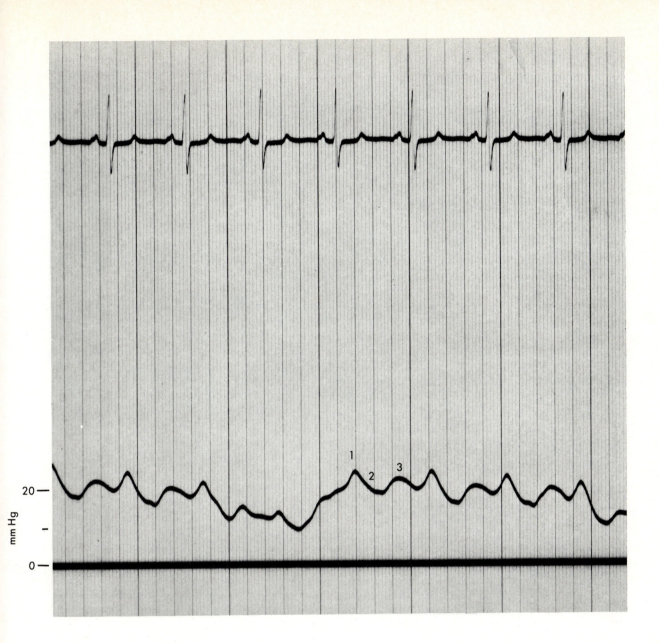

ANALYSIS

Rhythm: NSR

Pressure(s): PAW

Waveform characteristics and measurements:

1. _____ *a* Wave _____ ; _____ 21 _____ mm Hg

2. _____ *x* Descent _____ ; _____ mm Hg

3. _____ *v* Wave _____ ; _____ 20 _____ mm Hg

4. _____ Mean _____ ; _____ 19 _____ mm Hg

5. _____ ; _____ mm Hg

6. _____ ; _____ mm Hg

7. _____ ; _____ mm Hg

Suspected abnormality: CHF

Comments: Note the marked time delay between the electrical and corresponding mechanical event. This is likely due to increased catheter and tubing length.

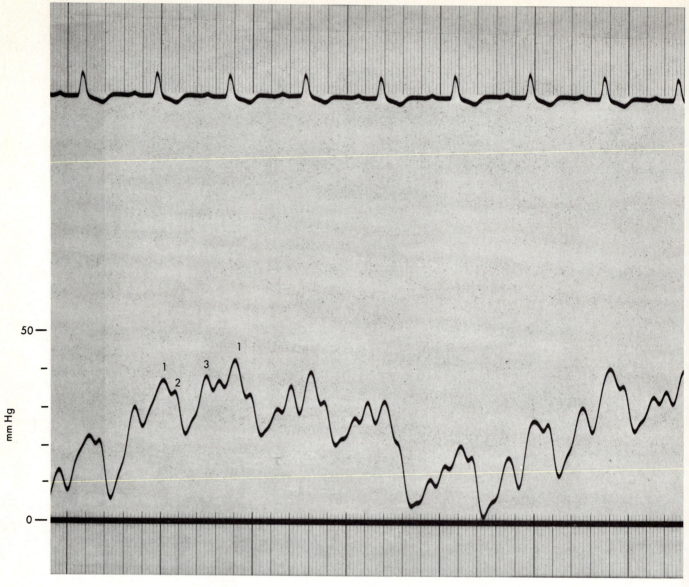

ANALYSIS

Rhythm: NSR

Pressure(s): PAW

Waveform characteristics and measurements:

1.	*a* Wave	;	30	mm Hg
2.	*c* Wave	;		mm Hg
3.	*v* Wave	;	27	mm Hg
4.	Mean	;	20	mm Hg
5.		;		mm Hg
6.		;		mm Hg
7.		;		mm Hg

Suspected abnormality: CHF

Comments: Note the slightly prominent *a* wave due to the prolonged PR interval. There is an exaggerated respiratory response in this PAW pressure tracing, making accurate calculation somewhat difficult. The measured values reflect the average pressures.

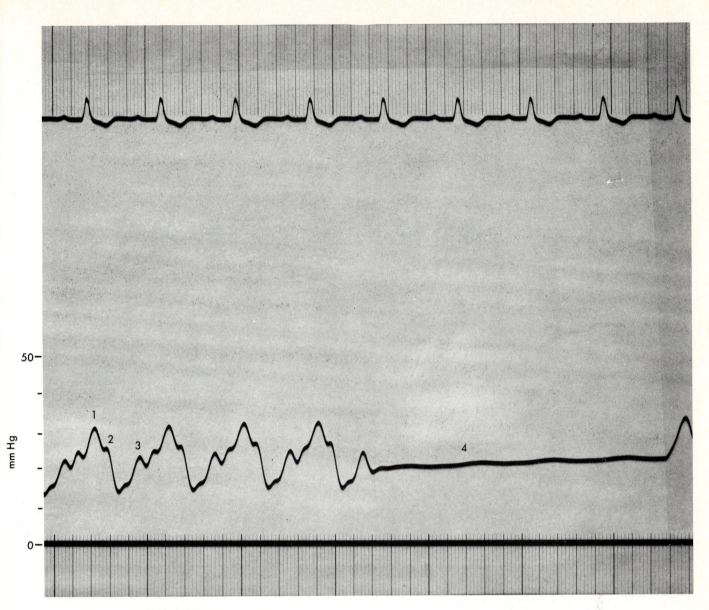

ANALYSIS

Rhythm: NSR

Pressure(s): PAW

Waveform characteristics and measurements:

1.	_a_ Wave	;	30	mm Hg
2.	_c_ Wave	;		mm Hg
3.	_v_ Wave	;	25	mm Hg
4.	Electrical mean	;	20	mm Hg
5.		;		mm Hg
6.		;		mm Hg
7.		;		mm Hg

Suspected abnormality: CHF

Comments: Comparison of this PAW with the PAW pressure waveform in Fig. 4-11 reveals a lack of respiratory variation while the patient momentarily suspends respirations at the end of the expiratory phase.

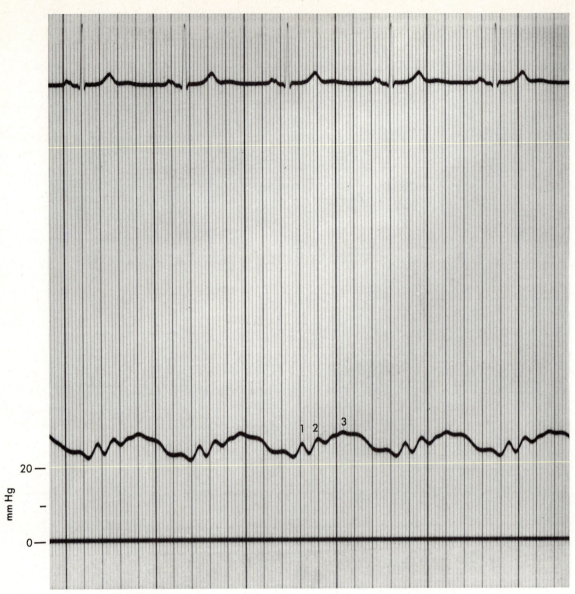

ANALYSIS

Rhythm: NSR

Pressure(s): PAW

Waveform characteristics and measurements:

1.	*a* Wave	;	25	mm Hg
2.	*c* Wave	;		mm Hg
3.	*v* Wave	;	27	mm Hg
4.	Mean	;	26	mm Hg
5.		;		mm Hg
6.		;		mm Hg
7.		;		mm Hg

Suspected abnormality: CHF

Comments: This PAW pressure waveform has a damped appearance but is clearly elevated, suggesting CHF.

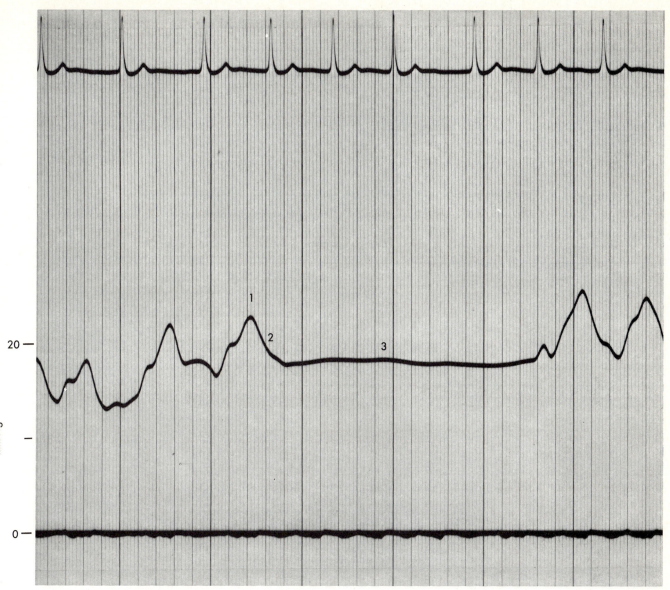

mm Hg

20 —

0 —

ANALYSIS

Rhythm: Atrial fibrillation

Pressure(s): PAW

Waveform characteristics and measurements:

1.	*v* Wave	;	22	mm Hg
2.	*y* Descent	;		mm Hg
3.	Electrical mean	;	19	mm Hg
4.		;		mm Hg
5.		;		mm Hg
6.		;		mm Hg
7.		;		mm Hg

Suspected abnormality: Mild mitral regurgitation with mild CHF

Comments: The elevated *v* wave lasting all of systole suggests some mitral regurgitation, whereas the slow *y* descent raises the question of concomitant mitral
stenosis.

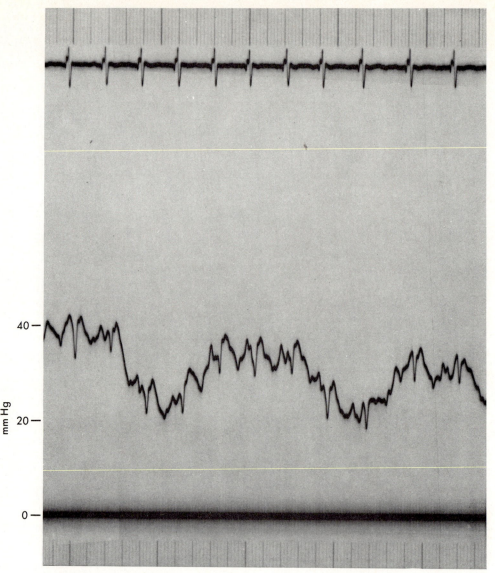

40 —

mm Hg

20 —

0 —

ANALYSIS

Rhythm: Atrial fibrillation

Pressure(s): PAW

Waveform characteristics and measurements:

1.	Mean	;	30	mm Hg
2.		;		mm Hg
3.		;		mm Hg
4.		;		mm Hg
5.		;		mm Hg
6.		;		mm Hg
7.		;		mm Hg

Suspected abnormality: CHF

Comments: There are no *a* waves in this PAW tracing because of atrial fibrillation. The rapid heart rate and numerous fibrillatory waves make identification of the *v* wave difficult. In this case, the mean PAW pressure is used to reflect LVedp.

76

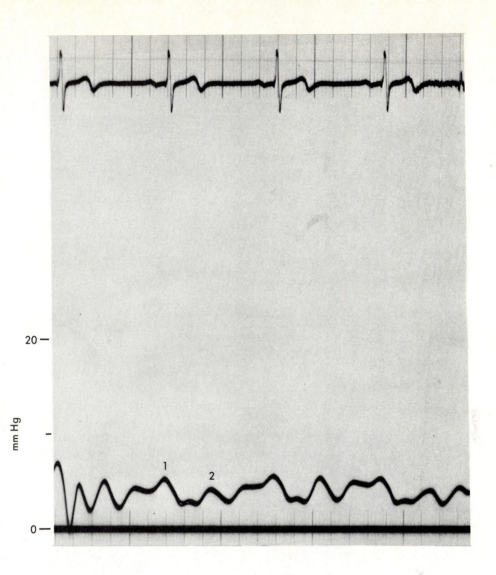

ANALYSIS

Rhythm: NSR

Pressure(s): PAW

Waveform characteristics and measurements:

1.	*a* Wave	;	5	mm Hg
2.	*v* Wave	;	5	mm Hg
3.	Mean	;	5	mm Hg
4.		;		mm Hg
5.		;		mm Hg
6.		;		mm Hg
7.		;		mm Hg

Suspected abnormality: Abnormally low PAW secondary to nitroprusside (Nipride) administration

Comments: Nitroprusside is a balanced venous and arterial vasodilator and therefore reduces both preload and afterload. During nitroprusside administration, particular attention must be given the PAW or PAedp to prevent reduction of the preload level to that point on the Starling ventricular function curve where cardiac output falls. Commonly, administration of volume during nitroprusside therapy is necessary to maintain an adequate preload level.

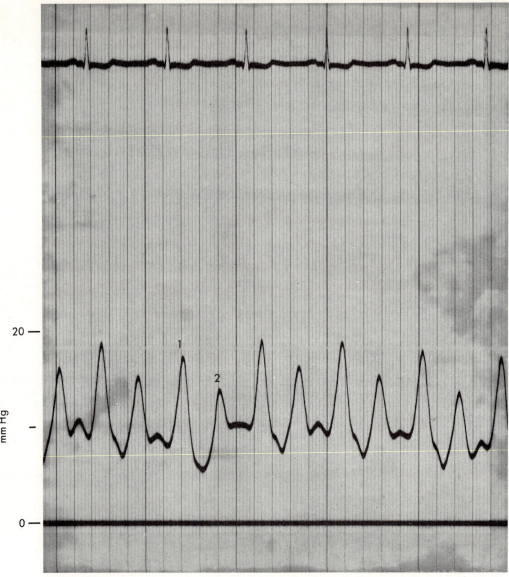

ANALYSIS

Rhythm: NSR

Pressure(s): PAW

Waveform characteristics and measurements:

1.	_a_ Wave	;	18 mm Hg
2.	_v_ Wave	;	15 mm Hg
3.	Mean	;	13 mm Hg
4.		;	mm Hg
5.		;	mm Hg
6.		;	mm Hg
7.		;	mm Hg

Suspected abnormality: LVH secondary to hypertension

Comments: Note the exaggerated _a_ wave due to left ventricular hypertrophy with decreased compliance during diastolic filling.

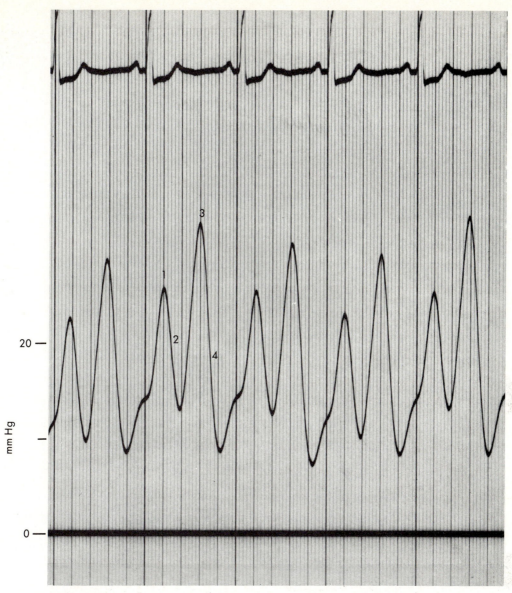

ANALYSIS

Rhythm: NSR

Pressure(s): PAW

Waveform characteristics and measurements:

1.	*a* Wave	;	26 mm Hg
2.	*x* Descent	;	mm Hg
3.	*v* Wave	;	32 mm Hg
4.	*y* Descent	;	mm Hg
5.		;	mm Hg
6.		;	mm Hg
7.		;	mm Hg

Suspected abnormality: LVH with mild mitral regurgitation

Comments: The elevated *a* wave of 26 mm Hg suggests resistance to LV filling, as in the case of LVH, where the ventricle becomes stiff and noncompliant. The elevated and dominant *v* wave indicates mitral regurgitation of mild severity.

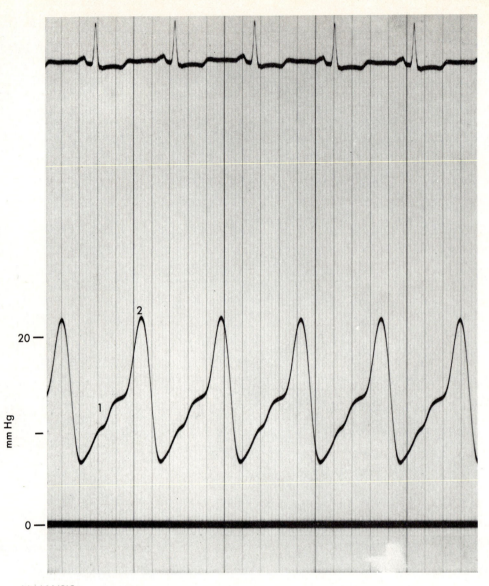

ANALYSIS

Rhythm: NSR

Pressure(s): PAW

Waveform characteristics and measurements:

1.	*a* Wave	;	10	mm Hg
2.	*v* Wave	;	22	mm Hg
3.		;		mm Hg
4.		;		mm Hg
5.		;		mm Hg
6.		;		mm Hg
7.		;		mm Hg

Suspected abnormality: Mild to moderate mitral regurgitation

Comments: The elevated, dominant *v* wave due to mitral regurgitation and blood flow into the left atrium during ventricular systole almost obscures the *a* wave in this PAW pressure waveform. However, the low value of the *a* wave (10 mm Hg) indicates that the left ventricle is performing well without any evidence of LV failure at this time.

80

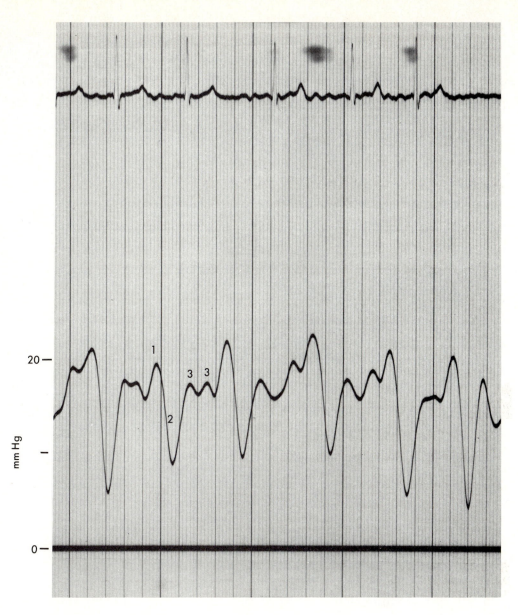

ANALYSIS

Rhythm: Atrial fibrillation

Pressure(s): PAW

Waveform characteristics and measurements:

1.	v wave	;	25 mm Hg
2.	y Descent	;	_____ mm Hg
3.	Possible fibrillation waves	;	_____ mm Hg
4.	_____	;	_____ mm Hg
5.	_____	;	_____ mm Hg
6.	_____	;	_____ mm Hg
7.	_____	;	_____ mm Hg

Suspected abnormality: CHF, possible mitral regurgitation

Comments: Note the elevated v wave and rapid y descent, suggestive of mitral regurgitation.

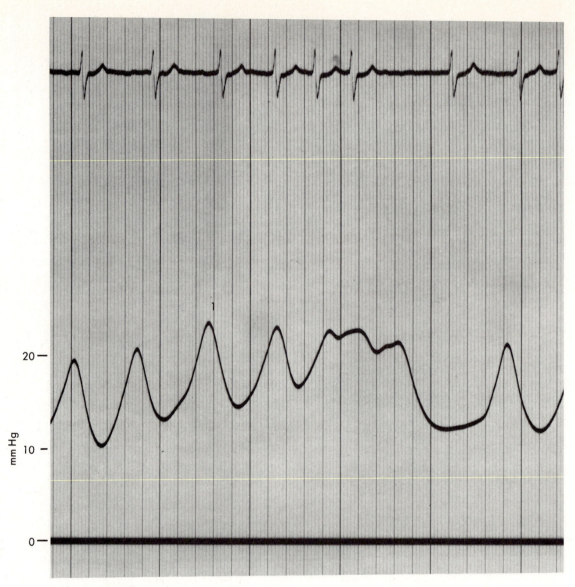

ANALYSIS

Rhythm: Atrial fibrillation

Pressure(s): PAW

Waveform characteristics and measurements:

1.	v Wave	;	22 mm Hg
2.	Mean	;	15 mm Hg
3.		;	mm Hg
4.		;	mm Hg
5.		;	mm Hg
6.		;	mm Hg
7.		;	mm Hg

Suspected abnormality: Mild to moderate mitral regurgitation

Comments: Note the effect of a three-beat run of tachycardia on the PAW pressure contour. This is due to the reduction in LV filling time, resulting in increased LA volume.

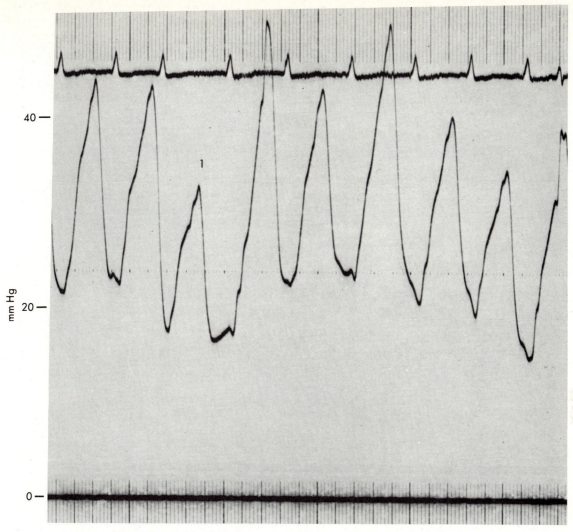

ANALYSIS

Rhythm: Atrial fibrillation

Pressure(s): PAW

Waveform characteristics and measurements:

1. _____ v Wave _____ ; _____ 48 _____ mm Hg

2. _____ ; _____ mm Hg

3. _____ ; _____ mm Hg

4. _____ ; _____ mm Hg

5. _____ ; _____ mm Hg

6. _____ ; _____ mm Hg

7. _____ ; _____ mm Hg

Suspected abnormality: Severe mitral regurgitation

Comments: A single v wave is seen corresponding with each QRS complex. The lack of a waves is due to atrial fibrillation. The elevated and dominant v wave is caused by mitral regurgitation with retrograde flow of blood into the left atrium during ventricular systole. Note the variation in the height of the v waves dependent on the RR interval and duration of LV filling. The third v wave is only about 30 mm Hg because of the short preceding RR interval and decreased filling of the LV. The fourth v wave, on the other hand, is markedly higher (52 mm Hg) because of the longer preceding RR interval and filling time of the LV.

83

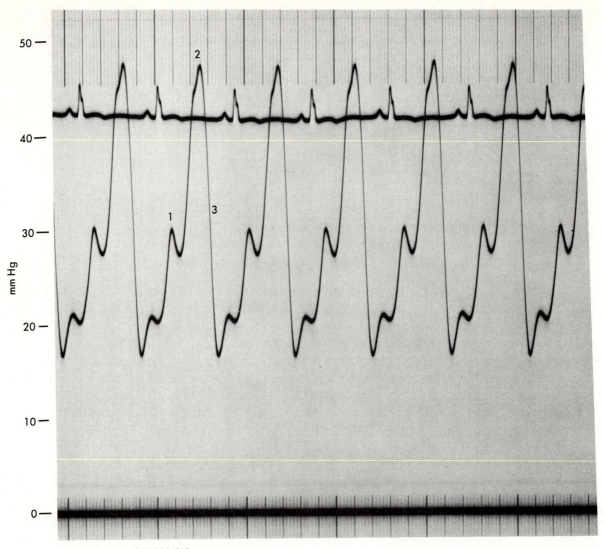

ANALYSIS

Rhythm: NSR

Pressure(s): PAW

Waveform characteristics and measurements:

1.	*a* Wave	;	30	mm Hg
2.	*v* Wave	;	48	mm Hg
3.	*y* Descent	;		mm Hg
4.		;		mm Hg
5.		;		mm Hg
6.		;		mm Hg
7.		;		mm Hg

Suspected abnormality: Mitral regurgitation with LV failure

Comments: The elevated and dominant *v* wave indicates mitral regurgitation, whereas the elevated *a* wave indicates LV failure. In this situation it is the PAW *a* wave that reflects LVedp, not the PAW mean pressure.

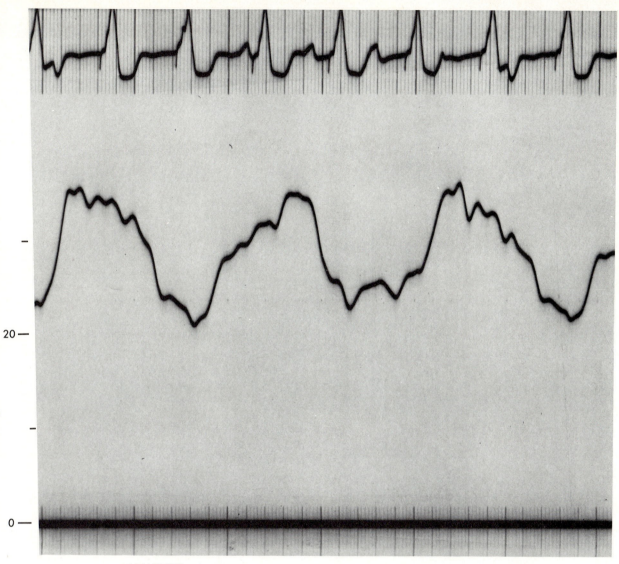

mm Hg

20 —

0 —

ANALYSIS

Rhythm: Paced (Note the pacemaker spikes and P waves throughout the ECG.)

Pressure(s): PAW

Waveform characteristics and measurements:

1. _____Mean_____ ; _____30_____ mm Hg
2. _____ ; _____ mm Hg
3. _____ ; _____ mm Hg
4. _____ ; _____ mm Hg
5. _____ ; _____ mm Hg
6. _____ ; _____ mm Hg
7. _____ ; _____ mm Hg

Suspected abnormality: Acute pulmonary edema

Comments: Such marked respiratory variation is commonly seen with acute pulmonary
edema or chronic obstructive pulmonary disease (COPD).

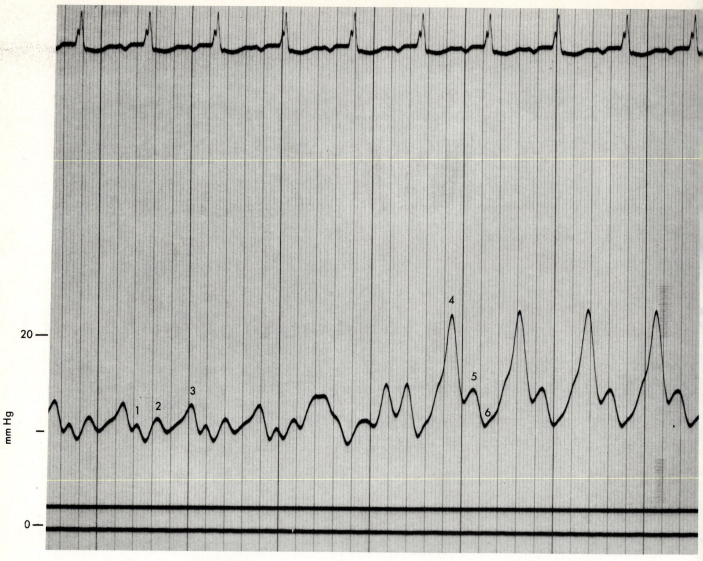

ANALYSIS

Rhythm: NSR

Pressure(s): PAW to PA

Waveform characteristics and measurements:

1.	PAW *a* wave	;	11	mm Hg
2.	PAW *c* wave	;		mm Hg
3.	PAW *v* wave	;	13	mm Hg
4.	PA systolic	;	24	mm Hg
5.	Dicrotic notch	;		mm Hg
6.	PA end-diastolic	;	11	mm Hg
7.		;		mm Hg

Suspected abnormality: Normal

Comments: The upstroke of this PA pressure waveform appears slightly damped, probably due to location of the catheter tip against the wall of the PA. Note the similarity between the PAW pressure and the PAedp. Once this correlation has been established, the PAedp can be used to monitor LVedp and thereby avoid frequent balloon inflations. Note the lack of respiratory variation as the patient momentarily suspends respirations at the end of expiration.

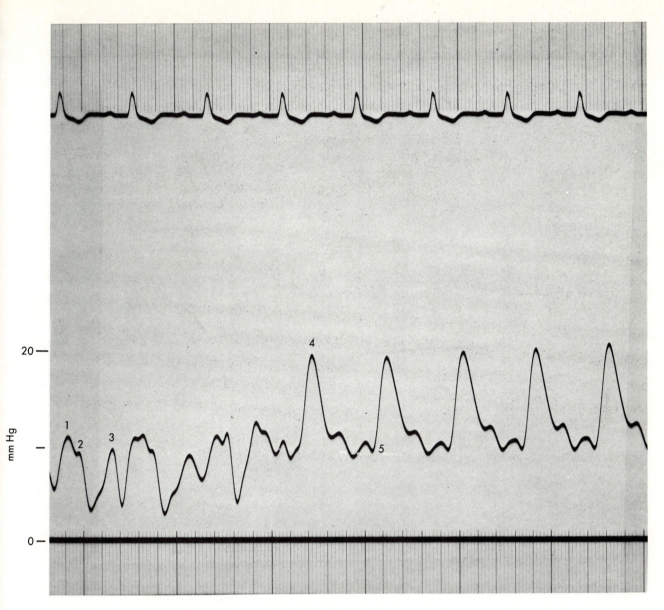

ANALYSIS

Rhythm: NSR

Pressure(s): PAW to PA

Waveform characteristics and measurements:

1.	PAW *a* wave	; 11	mm Hg
2.	PAW *c* wave	;	mm Hg
3.	PAW *v* wave	; 9	mm Hg
4.	PA systolic	; 20	mm Hg
5.	PA end-diastolic	; 10	mm Hg
6.		;	mm Hg
7.		;	mm Hg

Suspected abnormality: Normal

Comments: Note the correlation between PAW and PAedp.

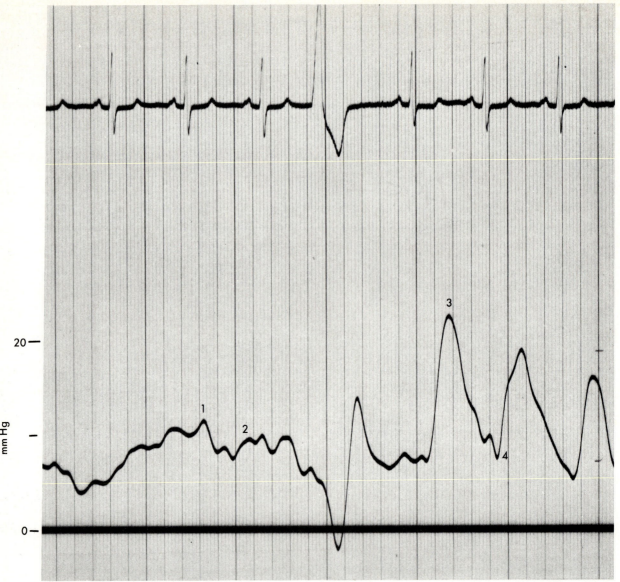

ANALYSIS

Rhythm: NSR with PVC

Pressure(s): PAW to PA

Waveform characteristics and measurements:

1.	PAW *a* wave	;	8	mm Hg
2.	PAW *v* wave	;	7	mm Hg
3.	PA systolic	;	18	mm Hg
4.	PA end-diastolic	;	8	mm Hg
5.		;		mm Hg
6.		;		mm Hg
7.		;		mm Hg

Suspected abnormality: Normal

Comments: Note the similarity between PAW and PAedp. Both pressures have a slightly damped appearance, which may be improved by aspiration and flushing of the distal lumen of the catheter while in the PA position.

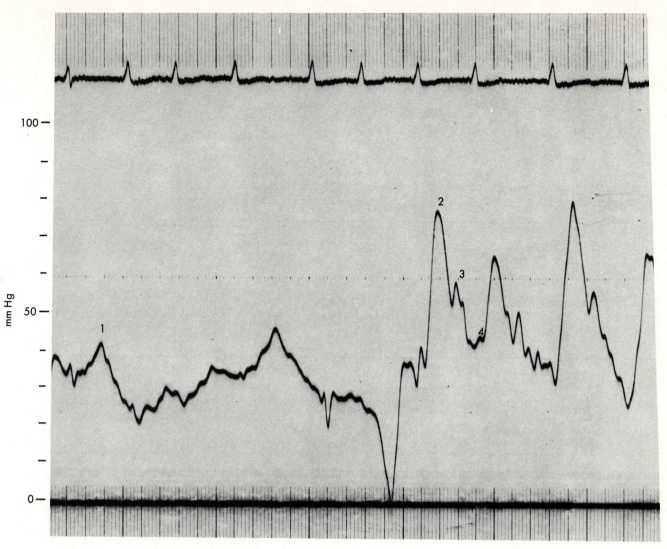

ANALYSIS

Rhythm: Atrial fibrillation

Pressure(s): PAW to PA

Waveform characteristics and measurements:

1.	PAW v wave	;	34	mm Hg
2.	PA systolic	;	70	mm Hg
3.	Dicrotic notch	;		mm Hg
4.	PA end-diastolic	;	35	mm Hg
5.		;		mm Hg
6.		;		mm Hg
7.		;		mm Hg

Suspected abnormality: Pulmonary hypertension secondary to severe CHF

Comments: Because of atrial fibrillation, there is only a v wave present in this somewhat damped PAW pressure waveform. Although there is considerable respiratory variation, the PAW v wave averages approximately 34 mm Hg, indicating severe CHF. Note the close correlation between the PAW mean and the PAedp.

89

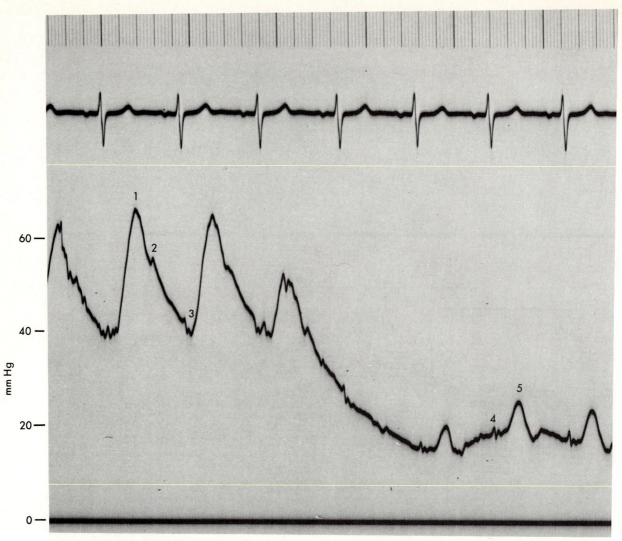

ANALYSIS

Rhythm: NSR

Pressure(s): PA to PAW

Waveform characteristics and measurements:

1.	PA systolic	;	65	mm Hg
2.	Dicrotic notch	;		mm Hg
3.	PA end-diastolic	;	40	mm Hg
4.	PAW *a* wave	;	18	mm Hg
5.	PAW *v* wave	;	21	mm Hg
6.		;		mm Hg
7.		;		mm Hg

Suspected abnormality: Pulmonary hypertension secondary to COPD with mild LV failure

Comments: Note the disparity between the PAedp and PAW pressure. This pulmonary hypertension is due to lung disease and does not reflect the LVedp. The PAW pressure, however, does reflect the LVedp and reveals mild LV failure (18 mm Hg) and perhaps a very small amount of mitral regurgitation secondary to LV dilatation.

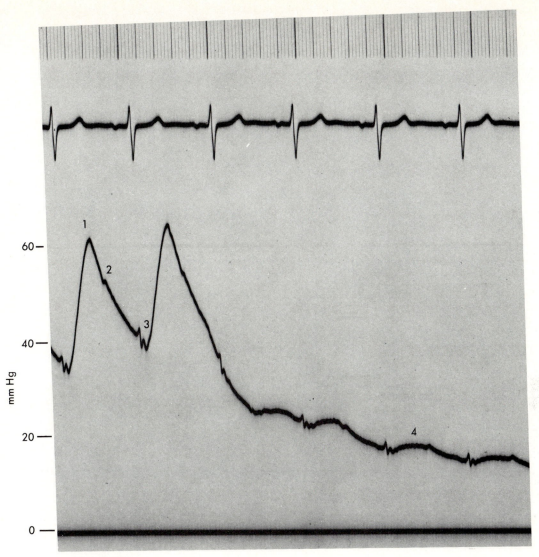

ANALYSIS

Rhythm: NSR

Pressure(s): PA to PAW

Waveform characteristics and measurements:

1.	PA systolic	;	60 mm Hg
2.	Dicrotic notch	;	mm Hg
3.	PA end-diastolic	;	37 mm Hg
4.	PAW mean	;	18 mm Hg
5.		;	mm Hg
6.		;	mm Hg
7.		;	mm Hg

Suspected abnormality: Pulmonary hypertension secondary to COPD with mild LV failure

Comments: These pressures are recorded from the same patient as on p. 90; however, these pressure waveforms are damped, making the accuracy of the pressure values questionable. Note particularly the lack of identifiable waves in the PAW pressure tracing. This catheter should be aspirated and flushed in the PA position before the recording of new pressures.

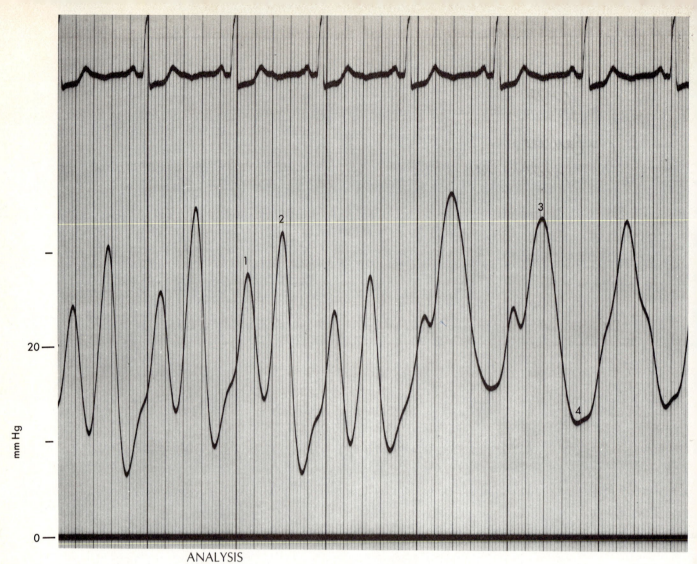

ANALYSIS

Rhythm: NSR

Pressure(s): PAW to PA

Waveform characteristics and measurements:

1.	PAW *a* wave	;	26	mm Hg
2.	PAW *v* wave	;	31	mm Hg
3.	PA systolic	;	33	mm Hg
4.	PA end-diastolic	;	15	mm Hg
5.		;		mm Hg
6.		;		mm Hg
7.		;		mm Hg

Suspected abnormality: Mild mitral regurgitation with mild CHF

Comments: Deflation of the balloon results in a distinct change in the PAW pressure. However, the PA pressure waveform is not of the usual PA pressure contour consisting of systole, dicrotic notch, and diastole. Additionally, the PAedp does not approximate the PAW pressure, suggesting a spurious PA pressure. The last four waveforms probably represent mixed PA/PAW pressure due to the distal location of the Swan-Ganz catheter tip. Slight withdrawal of the catheter could improve this problem. Confirmation of location of the catheter tip in either the PA or PAW position can be obtained by noting or measuring the oxygen saturation of a withdrawn blood sample. If the catheter tip is in the PA, the blood sample will have a venous saturation (<75%) and will have a dark appearance. If the catheter tip is truly wedged, obliterating forward flow, the blood sample will be arterialized (>90%), in the absence of pulmonary disease.

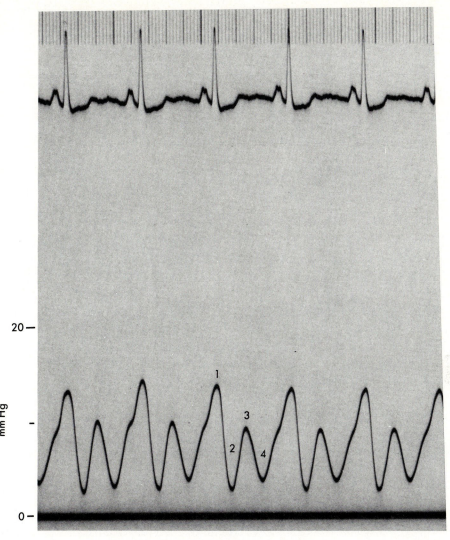

ANALYSIS

Rhythm: NSR

Pressure(s): LA

Waveform characteristics and measurements:

1.	*a* Wave	;	14 mm Hg
2.	*x* Descent	;	mm Hg
3.	*v* Wave	;	10 mm Hg
4.	Mean	;	9 mm Hg
5.		;	mm Hg
6.		;	mm Hg
7.		;	mm Hg

Suspected abnormality: Probably normal

Comments: Note the lack of respiratory response due to momentarily suspended respirations.

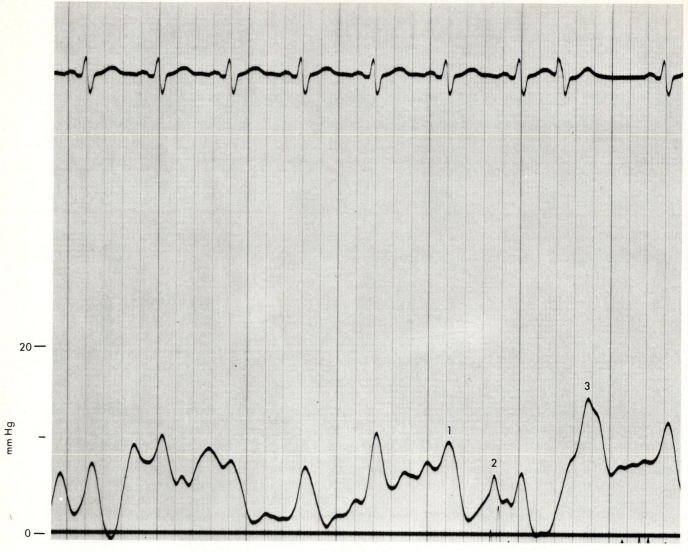

ANALYSIS

Rhythm: NSR with premature beat

Pressure(s): LA

Waveform characteristics and measurements:

1.	*a* Wave	;	9 mm Hg
2.	*v* Wave	;	9 mm Hg
3.	*v* Wave 2⁰ PB	;	mm Hg
4.	Mean	;	6 mm Hg
5.		;	mm Hg
6.		;	mm Hg
7.		;	mm Hg

Suspected abnormality: Normal

Comments: Note the large *v* wave that follows the premature beat. This is due to premature ventricular systole occurring at a time when the mitral valve is open.

94

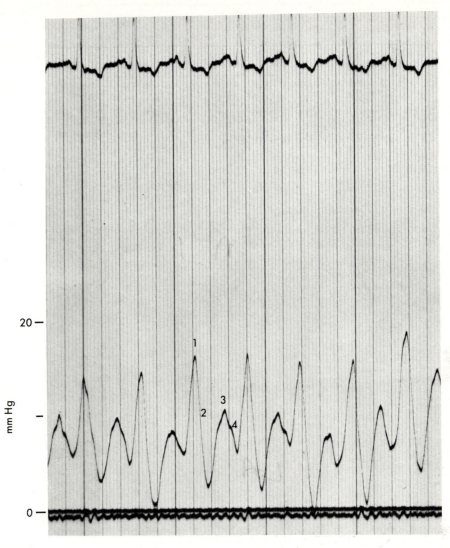

ANALYSIS

Rhythm: Sinus tachycardia

Pressure(s): LA

Waveform characteristics and measurements:

1. _____ *a* Wave _____ ; _____ 16 _____ mm Hg

2. _____ *x* Descent _____ ; _____ mm Hg

3. _____ *v* Wave _____ ; _____ 10 _____ mm Hg

4. _____ *y* Descent _____ ; _____ mm Hg

5. _____ ; _____ mm Hg

6. _____ ; _____ mm Hg

7. _____ ; _____ mm Hg

Suspected abnormality: LVH

Comments: The values of this LA pressure are normal, but the prominent *a* wave with rapid *x* descent suggests a stiff, hypertrophic LV.

chapter 5

Arterial pressures

Physiology and morphology

The arterial pressure waveform resembles the PA pressure waveform in contour, since the same physiologic events occur on the left side of the heart as on the right side of the heart. The value, however, is normally six times greater on the left side of the heart. The arterial pressure is divided into two phases: systole and diastole. Arterial systole begins with the opening of the aortic valve and rapid ejection of blood into the aorta. This is followed by runoff of blood from the proximal aorta to the peripheral arteries. On the arterial pressure waveform this is seen as a sharp rise in pressure followed by a decline in pressure. As the pressure falls, the aortic valve snaps shut, causing a small rise in arterial pressure that appears as a dip on the downslope and is termed the *dicrotic notch*. The *peak systolic pressure* (which reflects LV systolic pressure) is normally 100 to 140 mm Hg.

Diastole follows closure of the aortic valve and continues until the next systole. During this time, run-off to the peripheral arteries occurs without further flow from the LV. On the arterial pressure waveform this is seen as a gradual decrease in pressure. The lowest point of diastole (actually, end-diastole) is referred to as the *arterial diastolic pressure* and is normally 60 to 80 mm Hg.

The arterial pressure differs in both contour and value in various arterial locations. The systolic pressure is higher in the femoral artery than in the radial or brachial artery, by as much as 25 to 50 mm Hg. Generally, the diastolic values remain approximately the same. Additionally, the more distal the location of the arterial catheter, the sharper the upstroke and the less defined the dicrotic notch.

ECG correlation

The systolic arterial pressure rise occurs immediately following ventricular depolarization, i.e., after the QRS complex on the ECG. Again, there may be some delay, depending on the catheter location and length of tubing used. The dicrotic notch occurs after the T wave of the ECG.

In atrial fibrillation the arterial pressure value varies considerably (p. 103), depending on the RR intervals and length of time for ventricular filling.

When a PVC occurs, ventricular systole is initiated early, before the LV has had time to fill with blood. This results in a diminished stroke volume and lowered arterial pulse pressure. Isolated PVCs are usually well compensated for by a pause and an increase in stroke volume and arterial pressure with the succeeding contraction. Runs of PVCs, however, can be devastating, since there is virtually no opportunity for LV filling and, therefore stroke volume and arterial pressure fall precipitously (p. 111).

Abnormal findings

The arterial pressure is elevated in the following conditions:
1. Systemic hypertension
2. Arteriosclerosis
3. Aortic insufficiency

Additionally, certain drugs, including vasopressors and certain positive inotropic agents, can markedly increase arterial pressure by increasing systemic vascular resistance and/or increasing cardiac output.

The arterial pressure waveform with aortic insufficiency classically reveals a wide pulse pressure with an elevated systolic pressure and a lowered diastolic pressure (p. 110). This is due to rapid ejection of a large stroke volume (the normal stroke volume plus the regurgitant volume), with regurgitation of blood across the incompetent aortic valve during diastole. Additionally, the dicrotic notch on the downslope of the arterial pressure is usually absent.

The arterial pressure may be abnormally low in the following conditions:
1. Low cardiac output
2. Aortic stenosis
3. Arrhythmias

Certain drugs, including vasodilators and certain calcium antagonists, can also decrease arterial blood pressure by decreasing systemic vascular resistance.

The contour of the arterial pressure waveform with low cardiac output or even the state of shock is normal, but the value is abnormally low. The pulse pressure is narrow due to the small stroke volume ejected each beat.

Both the contour and the value of the arterial pressure are altered with aortic stenosis. Because of the increased resistance to ejection of blood through the narrowed aortic valve orifice, the upstroke of the arterial pressure waveform is slow and appears to rise at an angle rather than straight up. Often the dicrotic notch is not well defined and may appear as a "bend" on the downslope of the arterial pressure waveform. This is caused by the stiff closing movement of diseased aortic valve leaflets, which does not produce a rise in pressure. The value of the arterial pressure is low with a narrow pulse pressure, indicating a low stroke volume. It should be mentioned here that the contour of a damped arterial waveform closely resembles the arterial waveform of aortic stenosis.

The effects of arrhythmias on the arterial pressure waveform are discussed under the ECG correlation section.

Abnormalities of the arterial pressure waveform may be due to mechanical causes of damping, fling, or whip or inaccurate zeroing or calibrating. Damping produces an arterial pressure waveform similar to that of aortic stenosis, i.e., a slow upstroke, rounded appearance, poorly defined dicrotic notch, and narrow pulse pressure. A clot at the tip of the catheter or lodging of the catheter tip against the vessel wall is usually the cause, and gentle flushing or repositioning of the catheter tip eliminates this problem. Fling or whip in the arterial pressure waveform may be due to excessive movement of the catheter tip (p. 106).

Inaccurate zeroing or calibration alters the value but not the contour of the arterial pressure waveform. Zeroing and calibration should be repeated if there is any question regarding the accuracy of the arterial pressure. Improper placement of the air reference stopcock also alters the value of the arterial pressure. Placement of the air reference stopcock above the level of the RA results in an artifactually low pressure, whereas placement below the level of the RA results in an artifactually high pressure. This frequently is the problem if the patient's position has been changed.

Vasodilators (including certain calcium antagonists) affect both the contour and the value of the arterial pressure waveform. The decreased systemic vascular resistance and impedance to flow during afterload reduction cause a rapid upstroke of the arterial systolic pressure, a rapid decline in systolic pressure during the shorter ejection phase, and less change in pressure during diastole (the period of resistance-reduced runoff). The value of both the systolic and diastolic pressures are often reduced, although it is possible to greatly enhance the cardiac output and thereby cause little change in the arterial pressures.

Examples

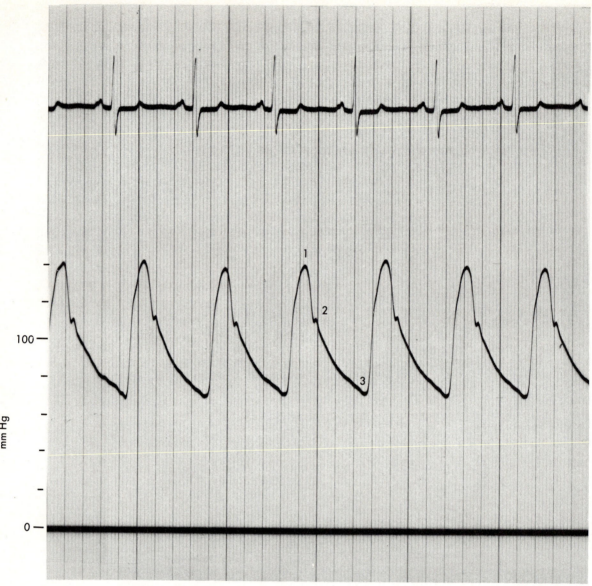

ANALYSIS

Rhythm: NSR

Pressure(s): Radial artery

Waveform characteristics and measurements:

1.	Arterial systolic	;	140	mm Hg
2.	Dicrotic notch	;		mm Hg
3.	Arterial end-diastolic	;	72	mm Hg
4.		;		mm Hg
5.		;		mm Hg
6.		;		mm Hg
7.		;		mm Hg

Suspected abnormality: Normal

Comments:

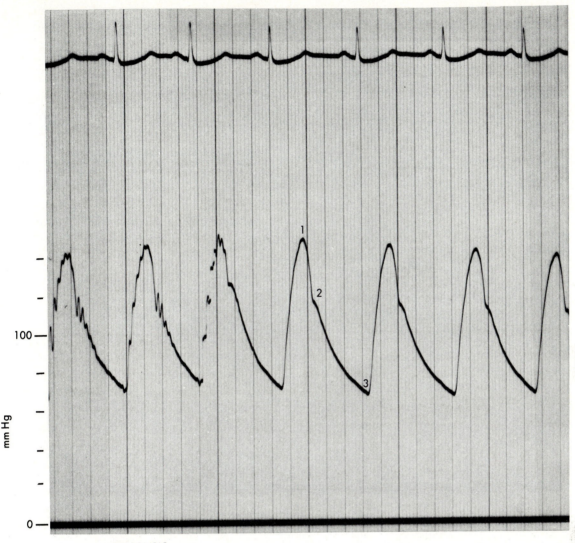

ANALYSIS

Rhythm: NSR

Pressure(s): Central arterial

Waveform characteristics and measurements:

1.	Arterial systolic	;	140	mm Hg
2.	Dicrotic notch	;		mm Hg
3.	Arterial end-diastolic	;	70	mm Hg
4.		;		mm Hg
5.		;		mm Hg
6.		;		mm Hg
7.		;		mm Hg

Suspected abnormality: Normal

Comments: Note the noise in the first three pressure waveforms due to catheter fling. This is resolved in the next four pressure waveforms by slight manipulation of the catheter.

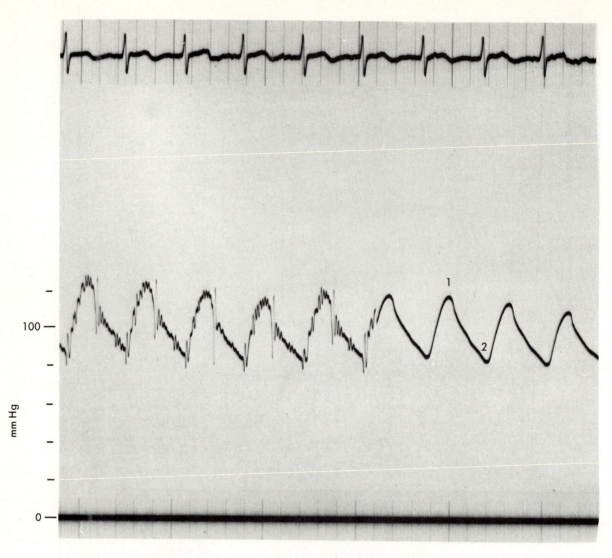

ANALYSIS

Rhythm: NSR

Pressure(s): Central arterial

Waveform characteristics and measurements:

1.	Arterial systolic	;	120 mm Hg
2.	Arterial end-diastolic	;	82 mm Hg
3.		;	mm Hg
4.		;	mm Hg
5.		;	mm Hg
6.		;	mm Hg
7.		;	mm Hg

Suspected abnormality: Normal

Comments: Note the presence of noise or fling in the first five pressure waveforms. It disappears in the last four pressure waveforms due to repositioning of the catheter tip. The contour actually becomes damped in appearance, probably due to placement of the catheter tip against the wall of the vessel. This produces a rounded-out appearance and lack of defined dicrotic notch.

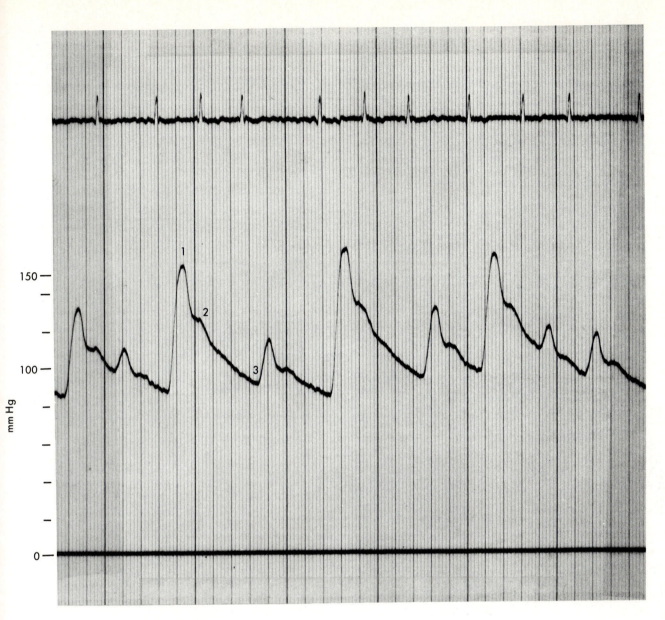

ANALYSIS

Rhythm: Atrial fibrillation

Pressure(s): Radial artery

Waveform characteristics and measurements:

1.	Arterial systolic	;	110-155	mm Hg
2.	Dicrotic notch	;		mm Hg
3.	Arterial end-diastolic	;	85	mm Hg
4.		;		mm Hg
5.		;		mm Hg
6.		;		mm Hg
7.		;		mm Hg

Suspected abnormality: Normal

Comments: Note the beat-to-beat variation in the arterial systolic pressure due to varying RR intervals with atrial fibrillation.

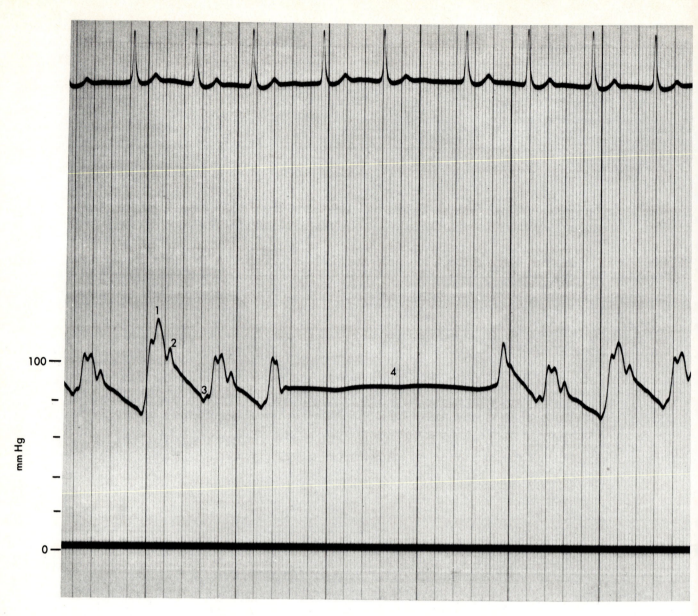

ANALYSIS

Rhythm: Atrial fibrillation

Pressure(s): Radial artery

Waveform characteristics and measurements:

#				
1.	Arterial systolic	;	99	mm Hg
2.	Dicrotic notch	;		mm Hg
3.	Arterial end-diastolic	;	70	mm Hg
4.	Electrical mean	;	80	mm Hg
5.		;		mm Hg
6.		;		mm Hg
7.		;		mm Hg

Suspected abnormality: Hypotension

Comments: Note the beat-to-beat variation due to varied RR intervals in atrial fibrillation. Note also how much closer the mean arterial pressure is to the diastolic pressure than to the systolic pressure.

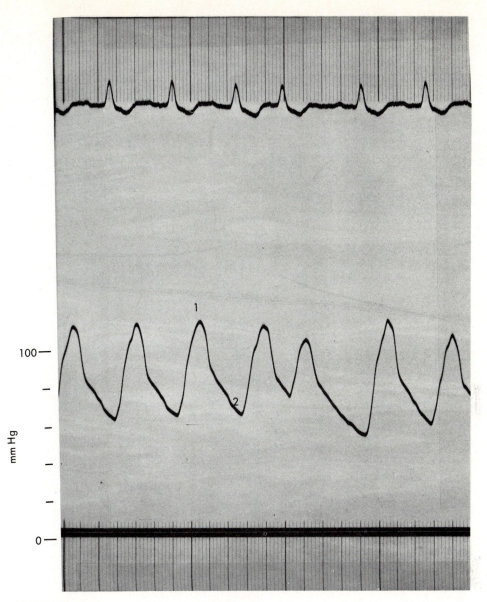

ANALYSIS

Rhythm: First-degree AV block with supraventricular beat

Pressure(s): Radial artery

Waveform characteristics and measurements:

1.	Arterial systolic	;	110	mm Hg
2.	Arterial end-diastolic	;	65	mm Hg
3.		;		mm Hg
4.		;		mm Hg
5.		;		mm Hg
6.		;		mm Hg
7.		;		mm Hg

Suspected abnormality: Normal

Comments: The damped quality of this arterial pressure waveform is evidenced by a rounded-out appearance and lack of sharp definition of the dicrotic notch. Aspiration and flushing will usually remedy this problem.

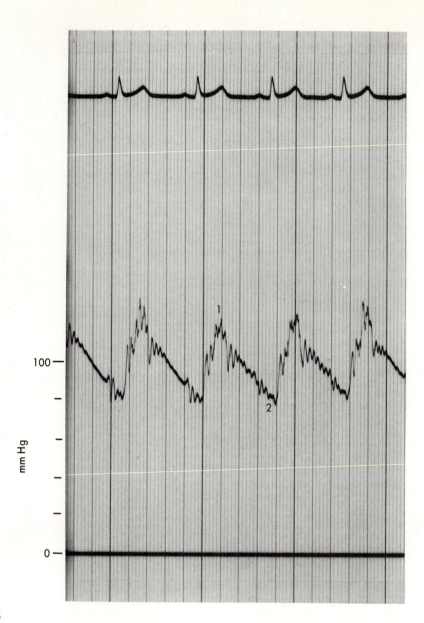

ANALYSIS

Rhythm: NSR

Pressure(s): Central arterial

Waveform characteristics and measurements:

1.	Arterial systolic	;	110 mm Hg
2.	Arterial end-diastolic	;	80 mm Hg
3.		;	mm Hg
4.		;	mm Hg
5.		;	mm Hg
6.		;	mm Hg
7.		;	mm Hg

Suspected abnormality: Normal

Comments: Note catheter fling due to turbulence met at the catheter tip in the central aorta.

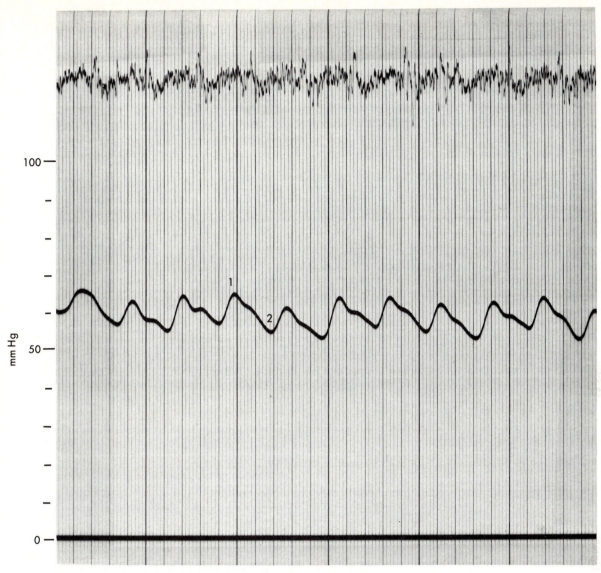

ANALYSIS

Rhythm: NSR (Note ECG interference.)

Pressure(s): Radial artery

Waveform characteristics and measurements:

1.	Arterial systolic	; 68	mm Hg
2.	Arterial end-diastolic	; 55	mm Hg
3.		;	mm Hg
4.		;	mm Hg
5.		;	mm Hg
6.		;	mm Hg
7.		;	mm Hg

Suspected abnormality: Severe hypotension

Comments: This arterial pressure waveform is very damped, showing a rounded-out contour, slow upstroke, and diminished pulse pressure. Aspiration and flushing usually alleviate this problem.

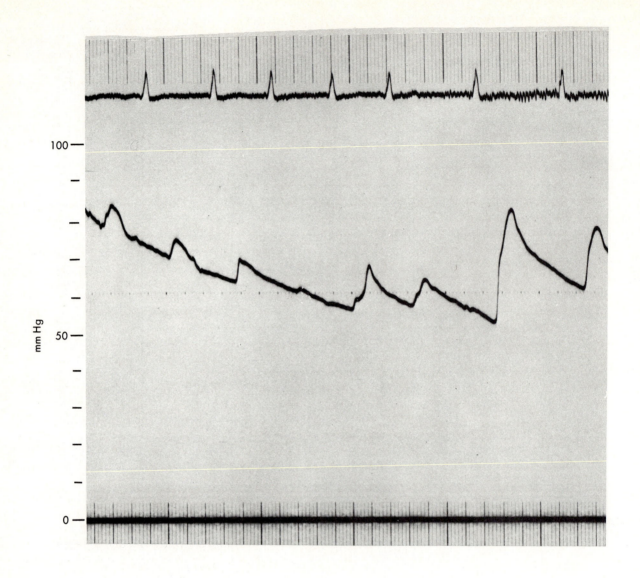

ANALYSIS

Rhythm: Atrial fibrillation

Pressure(s): (?) Possibly arterial

Waveform characteristics and measurements:

1. _____ ; _____ mm Hg

2. _____ ; _____ mm Hg

3. _____ ; _____ mm Hg

4. _____ ; _____ mm Hg

5. _____ ; _____ mm Hg

6. _____ ; _____ mm Hg

7. _____ ; _____ mm Hg

Suspected abnormality:

Comments: The stopcock from the patient to the transducer is only partially open.

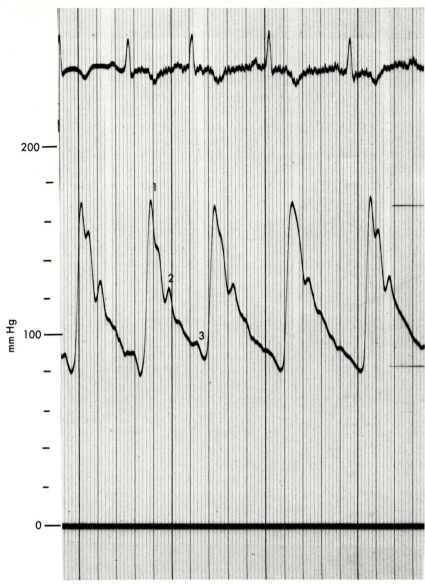

ANALYSIS

Rhythm: NSR

Pressure(s): Femoral artery

Waveform characteristics and measurements:

1.	Arterial systolic	;	170 mm Hg
2.	Dicrotic notch	;	_____ mm Hg
3.	Arterial end-diastolic	;	80 mm Hg
4.	_____	;	_____ mm Hg
5.	_____	;	_____ mm Hg
6.	_____	;	_____ mm Hg
7.	_____	;	_____ mm Hg

Suspected abnormality: Systolic hypertension secondary to arteriosclerosis

Comments:

109

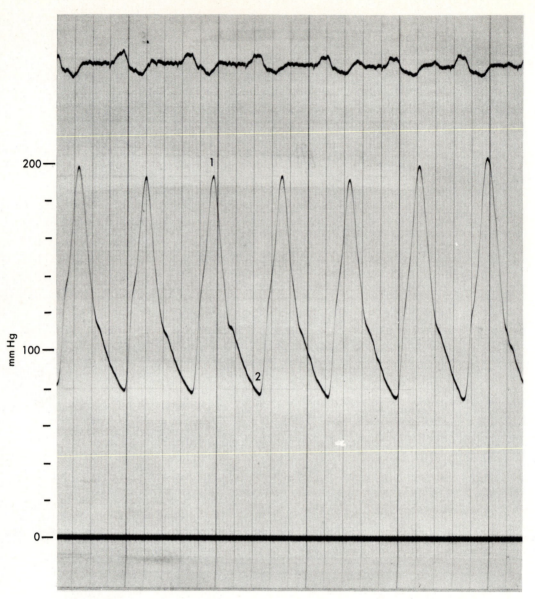

ANALYSIS

Rhythm: Paced (Note P waves throughout the ECG.)

Pressure(s): Radial artery

Waveform characteristics and measurements:

1.	Arterial systolic	;	200	mm Hg
2.	Arterial end-diastolic	;	80	mm Hg
3.		;		mm Hg
4.		;		mm Hg
5.		;		mm Hg
6.		;		mm Hg
7.		;		mm Hg

Suspected abnormality: Aortic regurgitation

Comments: Note the wide pulse pressure (120 mm Hg) and ill-defined dicrotic notch.

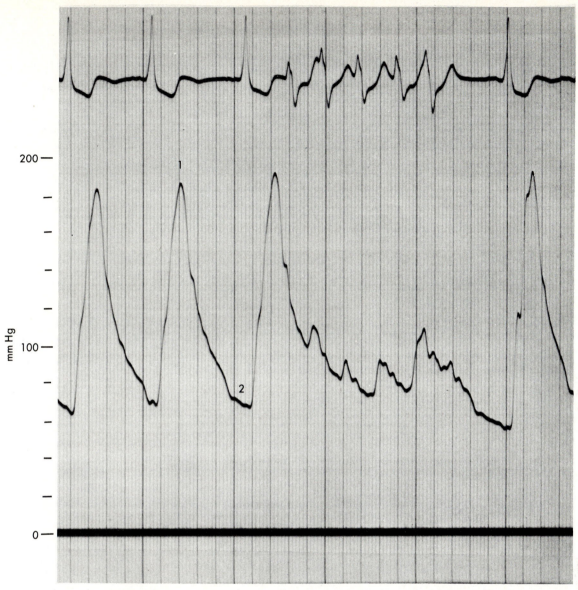

ANALYSIS

Rhythm: NSR with five-beat run of PVCs

Pressure(s): Radial artery

Waveform characteristics and measurements:

1.	Arterial systolic	;	180	mm Hg
2.	Arterial end-diastolic	;	60	mm Hg
3.		;		mm Hg
4.		;		mm Hg
5.		;		mm Hg
6.		;		mm Hg
7.		;		mm Hg

Suspected abnormality: Aortic regurgitation

Comments: Note the wide pulse pressure (120 mm Hg) and poorly defined or absent dicrotic notch, indicative of aortic regurgitation. Note also the devastating effects of a five-beat run of VT with a drop in arterial pressure to approximately 60 mm Hg, with minimal stroke volume.

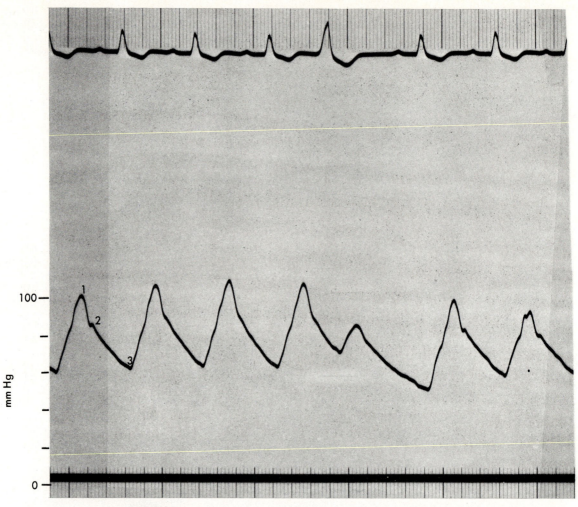

ANALYSIS

Rhythm: NSR with PVC

Pressure(s): Radial artery

Waveform characteristics and measurements:

1.	Arterial systolic	;	92	mm Hg
2.	Dicrotic notch	;		mm Hg
3.	Arterial end-diastolic	;	60	mm Hg
4.		;		mm Hg
5.		;		mm Hg
6.		;		mm Hg
7.		;		mm Hg

Suspected abnormality: Aortic stenosis

Comments: The slow upstroke of the arterial pulse is seen in aortic stenosis due to the resistance to ejection at the aortic valve. The poorly defined dicrotic notch is due to stiff movement and closure of the aortic valve leaflets. Additionally, the narrow pulse pressure indicates a small stroke volume due to aortic stenosis. Note the even further decrease in pressure and stroke volume following a premature ventricular beat, which reduced the amount of time for LV filling.

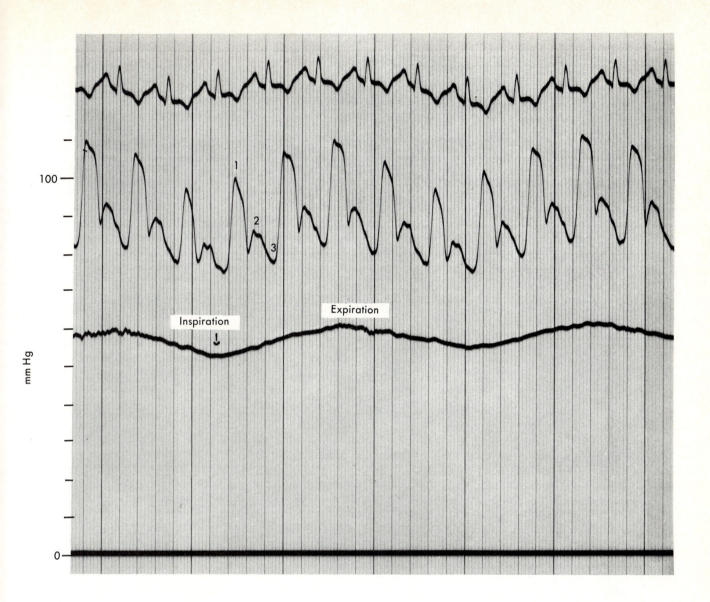

ANALYSIS

Rhythm: Sinus tachycardia

Pressure(s): Radial artery

Waveform characteristics and measurements:

1.	Arterial systolic	96-110	mm Hg
2.	Dicrotic notch		mm Hg
3.	Arterial end-diastolic	65-70	mm Hg
4.			mm Hg
5.			mm Hg
6.			mm Hg
7.			mm Hg

Suspected abnormality: Cardiac tamponade

Comments: Note the exaggerated decline in the arterial systolic pressure during inspiration (from 110 to 96 mm Hg). This is termed *paradoxical pulse* and occurs classically in cardiac tamponade. The physiologic mechanism producing this phenomenon is complex but is due, in part, to an inspiratory decrease in LV diastolic volume with a concomitant inspiratory decrease in LV stroke volume.

113

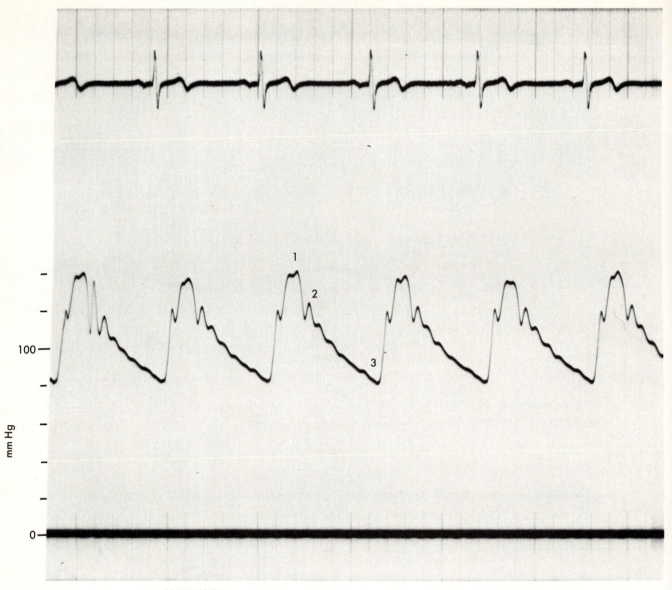

ANALYSIS

Rhythm: NSR

Pressure(s): Radial artery

Waveform characteristics and measurements:

1.	Arterial systolic	;	140	mm Hg
2.	Dicrotic notch	;		mm Hg
3.	Arterial end-diastolic	;	80	mm Hg
4.		;		mm Hg
5.		;		mm Hg
6.		;		mm Hg
7.		;		mm Hg

Suspected abnormality: Normal

Comments:

114

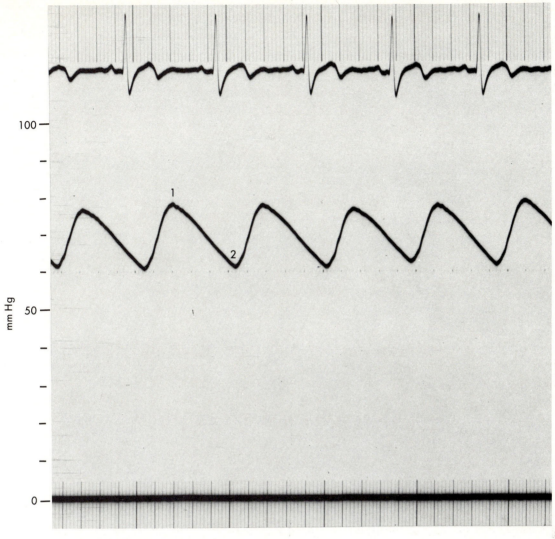

ANALYSIS

Rhythm: NSR

Pressure(s): Femoral artery

Waveform characteristics and measurements:

1.	Arterial systolic	;	77	mm Hg
2.	Arterial end-diastolic	;	60	mm Hg
3.		;		mm Hg
4.		;		mm Hg
5.		;		mm Hg
6.		;		mm Hg
7.		;		mm Hg

Suspected abnormality: Coarctation of the aorta or atherosclerosis of midabdominal aorta

Comments: Note the damped appearance of this arterial pressure waveform compared with this patient's radial artery pressure (p. 114), revealing a 65 mm Hg systolic gradient. This discrepancy is due to coarctation of the aorta. (Note that this arterial pressure is recorded on a different scale.)

115

chapter 6

Patient profiles

Invasive hemodynamic monitoring is used in a variety of clinical situations. It can be helpful in the diagnosis of certain pathologic conditions, such as pulmonary embolus or ventricular septal defect. (With pulmonary embolus the PAedp may be elevated, whereas the PAWm may be normal or low; with a VSD the oxygen saturation of a blood sample from the PA will be higher than an RA blood oxygen saturation.) Its major application, however, remains as a continuous assessment of the cardiovascular state of high-risk medical or surgical situations (myocardial infarction, openheart surgery, high-risk general surgery, ARDS, and burns). Hemodynamic data provide detailed, finely focused information that serves as an adjunct to the broader picture obtained through clinical assessment. Additionally, it offers a means of immediately evaluating the effectiveness or ineffectiveness of therapeutic interventions. Administration of certain pharmacologic agents can be carefully individualized and titrated according to the hemodynamic response.

This chapter provides nine patient profiles to illustrate the varied situations in which invasive hemodynamic monitoring is employed and the hemodynamic response to certain therapeutic agents. Additionally, it provides the opportunity for furthering skills in waveform identification and interpretation.

Patient profile 1

A 64-year-old man underwent triple coronary bypass surgery. At the time of surgery a Swan-Ganz and an arterial catheter were inserted. On the second postoperative day the patient developed atrial fibrillation. The following five pressure tracings were obtained at this time (pp. 119 to 123).

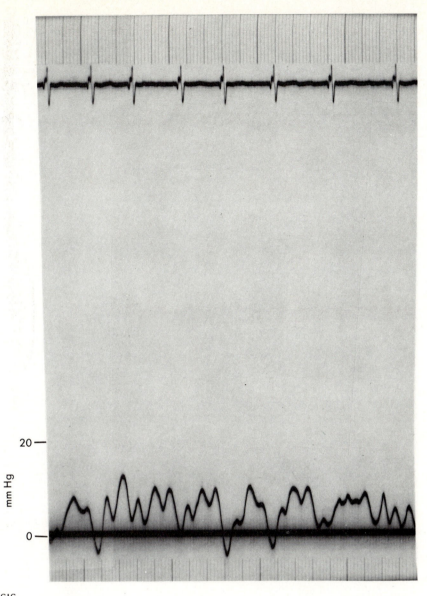

ANALYSIS

Rhythm: Atrial fibrillation

Pressure(s): RA

Waveform characteristics and measurements:

1. _____ Mean _____ ; _____ 7 _____ mm Hg

2. _____ ; _____ mm Hg

3. _____ ; _____ mm Hg

4. _____ ; _____ mm Hg

5. _____ ; _____ mm Hg

6. _____ ; _____ mm Hg

7. _____ ; _____ mm Hg

Suspected abnormality: Normal

Comments: The *a* waves are absent in this RA waveform due to atrial fibrillation. The *v* waves are difficult to discern from the fibrillatory waves present in this tracing. At any rate, the *v* wave is not dominant or markedly elevated.

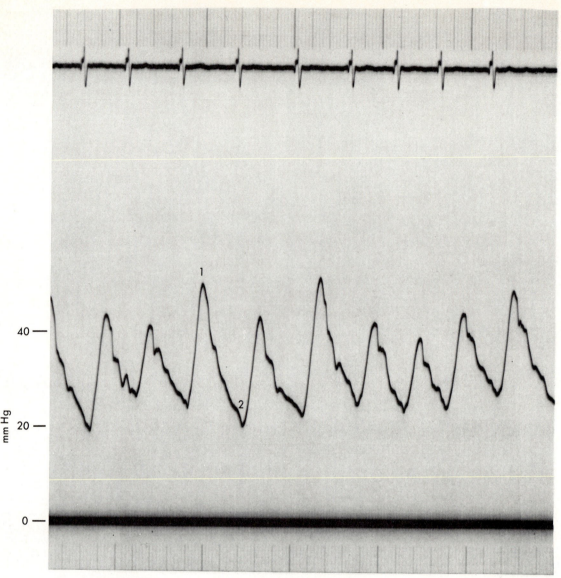

40 —

mm Hg

20 —

0 —

ANALYSIS

Rhythm: Atrial fibrillation

Pressure(s): PA

Waveform characteristics and measurements:

1.	PA systolic	; 45	mm Hg
2.	PA end-diastolic	; 22	mm Hg
3.		;	mm Hg
4.		;	mm Hg
5.		;	mm Hg
6.		;	mm Hg
7.		;	mm Hg

Suspected abnormality: CHF

Comments: Note the variation in peak PA systolic pressures due to both respiratory variation and changes in RR intervals and diastolic filling time. Note also the more elevated end-diastolic pressures when the ventricular response rate is faster.

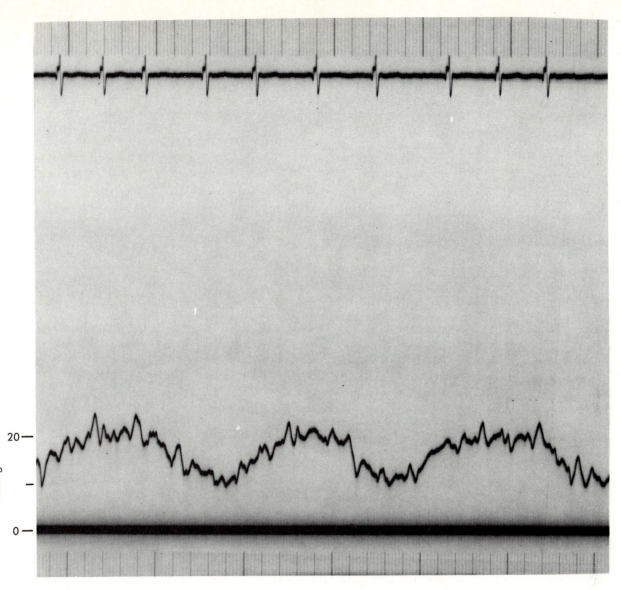

ANALYSIS

Rhythm: Atrial fibrillation

Pressure(s): PAW

Waveform characteristics and measurements:

1. _____Mean_____ ; _____18_____ mm Hg
2. _____ ; _____ mm Hg
3. _____ ; _____ mm Hg
4. _____ ; _____ mm Hg
5. _____ ; _____ mm Hg
6. _____ ; _____ mm Hg
7. _____ ; _____ mm Hg

Suspected abnormality: Mild CHF

Comments: Because the patient is in atrial fibrillation, there are no *a* waves in this PAW waveform. The *v* wave is difficult to discern because of the many fibrillatory waves in the waveform. However, it does not appear to be dominant or significantly elevated.

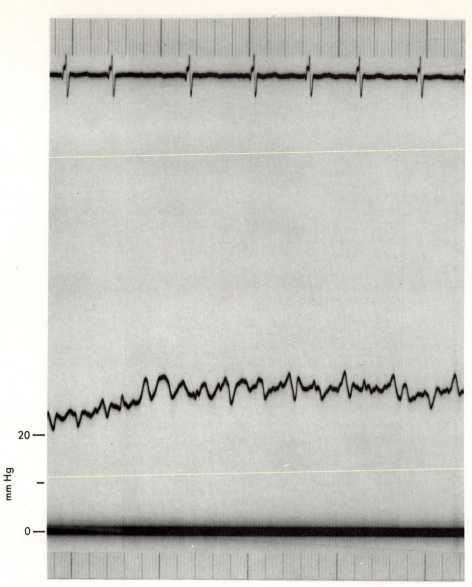

ANALYSIS

Rhythm: Atrial fibrillation

Pressure(s): PAW

Waveform characteristics and measurements:

1. _____No discernible waves_____ ; _____ mm Hg

2. _____ ; _____ mm Hg

3. _____ ; _____ mm Hg

4. _____ ; _____ mm Hg

5. _____ ; _____ mm Hg

6. _____ ; _____ mm Hg

7. _____ ; _____ mm Hg

Suspected abnormality: Overwedged pressure

Comments: Note the linearly rising appearance of this PAW pressure waveform. This is due to overdamping caused by overinflation or eccentric inflation of the balloon over the tip of the catheter.

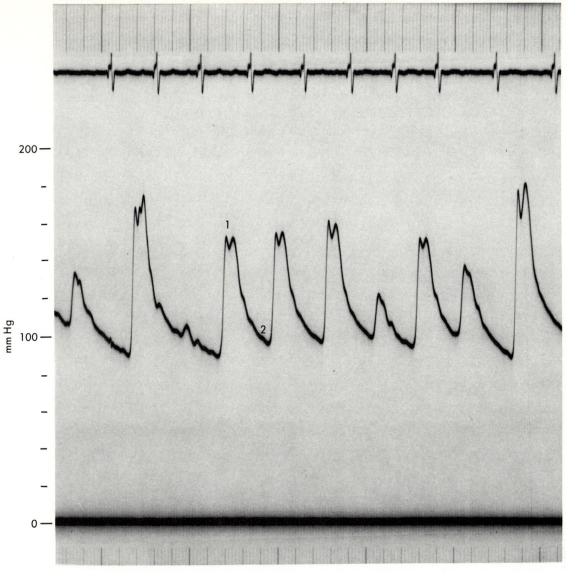

ANALYSIS

Rhythm: Atrial fibrillation

Pressure(s): Radial artery

Waveform characteristics and measurements:

1.	Arterial systolic	;	120-160	mm Hg
2.	Arterial end-diastolic	;	90	mm Hg
3.		;		mm Hg
4.		;		mm Hg
5.		;		mm Hg
6.		;		mm Hg
7.		;		mm Hg

Suspected abnormality: Normal

Comments: Note the variations in the arterial systolic values due to atrial fibrillation and the variable RR intervals affecting diastolic filling time.

123

Patient profile 2

A 59-year-old man was admitted to the CCU with evidence of an acute myocardial infarction, including ST and enzyme changes and rales. After 2 days of diuretic therapy, the patient became mildly hypotensive, raising the question of postdiuresis volume depletion. For this reason a Swan-Ganz catheter was inserted, and the following three hemodynamic pressure tracings were obtained (pp. 125 to 127), in addition to a cardiac index of 2.2 L/min/m^2.

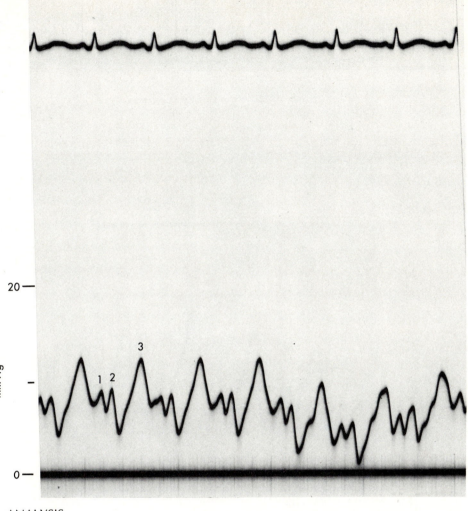

ANALYSIS

Rhythm: NSR

Pressure(s): PAW

Waveform characteristics and measurements:

1.	*a* Wave	;	7 mm Hg
2.	*c* Wave	;	mm Hg
3.	*v* Wave	;	10 mm Hg
4.	Mean	;	7 mm Hg
5.		;	mm Hg
6.		;	mm Hg
7.		;	mm Hg

Suspected abnormality: Hypovolemia secondary to diuresis

Comments: The lack of delay between electrical and mechanical events suggests that a miniature transducer was used without any extension tubing. Even though the contour and value of this PAW fall within the normal limits, in the presence of a low CI of 2.2 L/min/m², this filling pressure is too low to maintain adequate stroke volume. The reduction in volume following diuresis has placed the preload level lower on the ventricular function curve, reducing cardiac output.

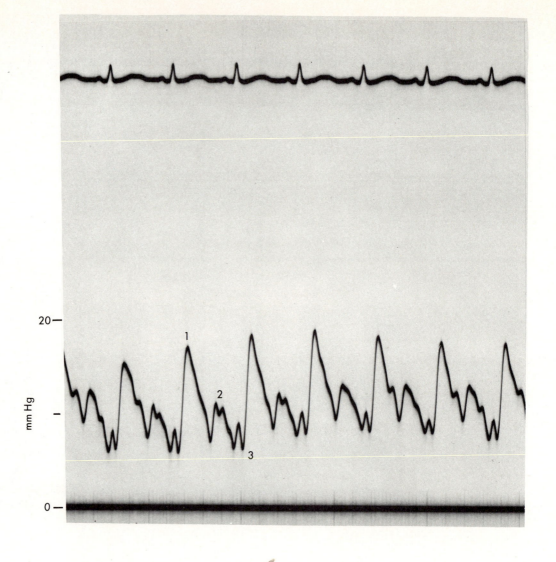

ANALYSIS

Rhythm: NSR

Pressure(s): PA

Waveform characteristics and measurements:

1.	PA systolic	;	19	mm Hg
2.	Retrograde LA *v* wave	;		mm Hg
3.	PA end-diastolic	;	8	mm Hg
4.		;		mm Hg
5.		;		mm Hg
6.		;		mm Hg
7.		;		mm Hg

Suspected abnormality: Hypovolemia secondary to diuresis

Comments: Note the close correlation between the PAedp and the PAW mean pressure shown on p. 125.

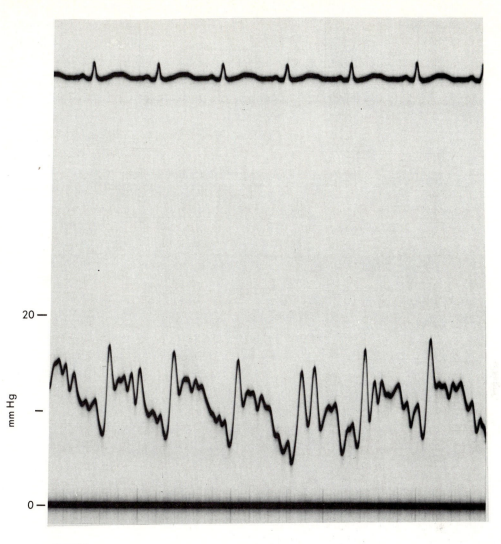

ANALYSIS

Rhythm: NSR

Pressure(s): Mixed PA/PAW

Waveform characteristics and measurements:

1. _____ ; _____ mm Hg

2. _____ ; _____ mm Hg

3. _____ ; _____ mm Hg

4. _____ ; _____ mm Hg

5. _____ _____ ; _____ mm Hg

6. _____ _____ ; _____ mm Hg

7. _____ ; _____ mm Hg

Suspected abnormality: Distal migration of the catheter tip

Comments: This supposed PA pressure waveform represents a mixed PA/PAW caused by distal migration of the catheter tip, resulting in partial occlusion of the vessel. Slight withdrawal of the catheter is necessary to safely monitor the PA pressure.

Patient profile 3

An 18-year-old man was admitted to the CCU with hypotension and symptoms of both right- and left-sided heart failure. A Swan-Ganz and an arterial catheter were inserted and revealed a cardiac index of 1.2 L/min/m^2 in addition to the following 5 hemodynamic pressure tracings (pp. 129 to 133).

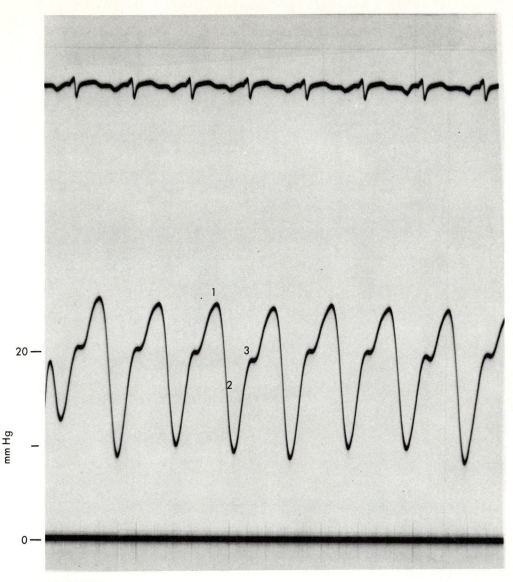

ANALYSIS

Rhythm: Sinus tachycardia

Pressure(s): RA

Waveform characteristics and measurements:

1.	*v* Wave	;	25	mm Hg
2.	*y* Descent	;		mm Hg
3.	*a* Wave	;	20	mm Hg
4.		;		mm Hg
5.		;		mm Hg
6.		;		mm Hg
7.		;		mm Hg

Suspected abnormality: RV failure with mild tricuspid regurgitation

Comments: The RA *v* wave is elevated and dominant with a rapid *y* descent, suggesting tricuspid regurgitation, probably functional and secondary to RV dilatation and failure. The elevated *a* wave indicates increased resistance to ventricular filling due to RV failure.

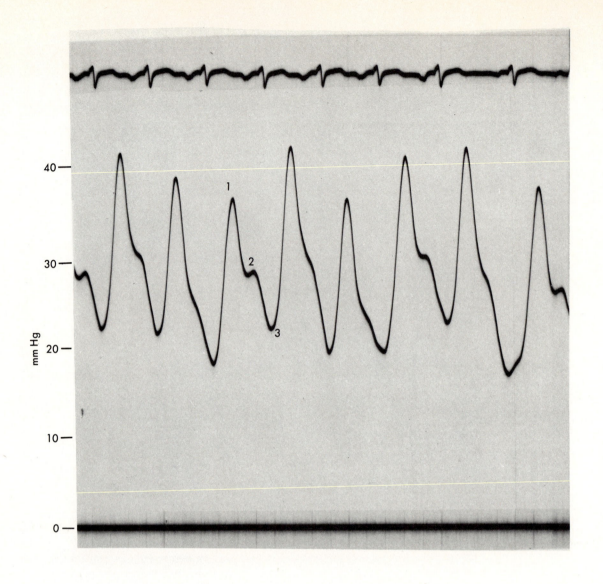

ANALYSIS

Rhythm: Sinus tachycardia

Pressure(s): PA

Waveform characteristics and measurements:

1.	PA systolic	;	40	mm Hg
2.	Dicrotic notch	;		mm Hg
3.	PA end-diastolic	;	23	mm Hg
4.		;		mm Hg
5.		;		mm Hg
6.		;		mm Hg
7.		;		mm Hg

Suspected abnormality: LV failure

Comments: Note the respiratory variation in the PA waveform with a rather rapid respiratory rate.

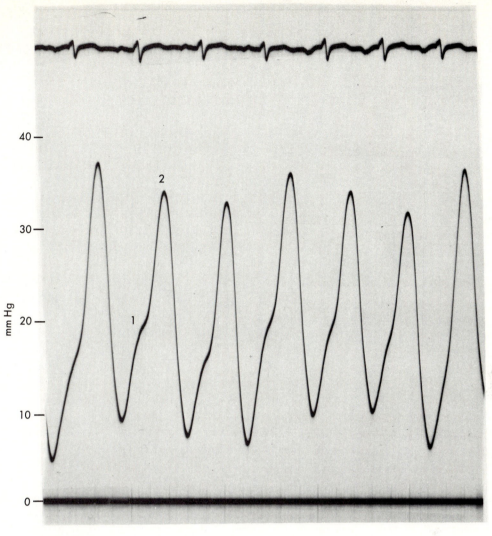

ANALYSIS

Rhythm: NSR

Pressure(s): PAW

Waveform characteristics and measurements:

1.	*a* Wave	;	20 mm Hg
2.	*v* Wave	;	37 mm Hg
3.	*y* Descent	;	mm Hg
4.		;	mm Hg
5.		;	mm Hg
6.		;	mm Hg
7.		;	mm Hg

Suspected abnormality: LV failure and mitral regurgitation secondary to papillary muscle dysfunction

Comments: The early, dominant, and elevated PAW *v* wave virtually obscures the PAW *a* wave. The rapid *y* descent following the large *v* wave is characteristic of mitral regurgitation and is due to the early, facile emptying of the left atrium. Note the correlation of the PAW *a* wave to the PAedp on p. 130.

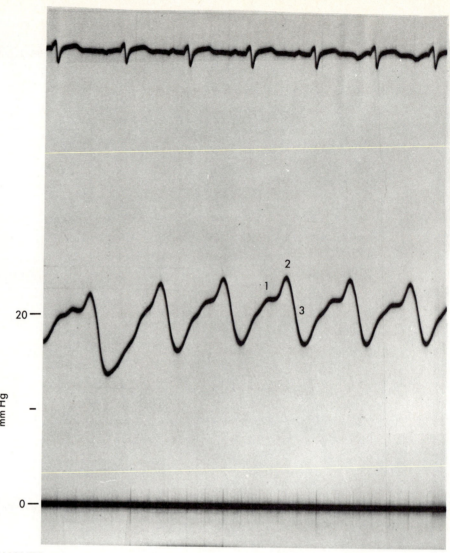

ANALYSIS

Rhythm: NSR

Pressure(s): PAW

Waveform characteristics and measurements:

1.	_a_ Wave	;	21	mm Hg
2.	_v_ Wave	;	25	mm Hg
3.	_y_ Descent	;		mm Hg
4.		;		mm Hg
5.		;		mm Hg
6.		;		mm Hg
7.		;		mm Hg

Suspected abnormality: CHF with mild to moderate mitral regurgitation

Comments: This patient was treated with nitroprusside in an attempt to increase forward flow and reduce the regurgitant volume. Compare this PAW pressure to the previous PAW pressure tracing (p. 131) and note the marked decrease in the _v_ wave from 35 to 26 mm Hg.

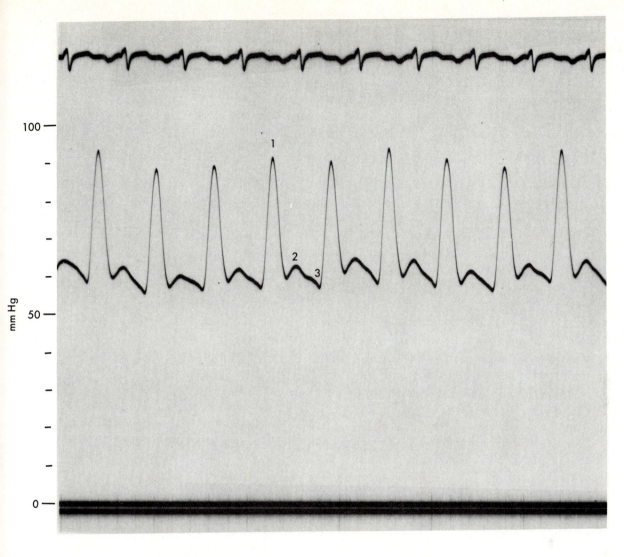

ANALYSIS

Rhythm: Sinus tachycardia

Pressure(s): Radial artery

Waveform characteristics and measurements:

1.	Peak systolic	;	92	mm Hg
2.	Dicrotic notch	;		mm Hg
3.	End-diastolic	;	55	mm Hg
4.		;		mm Hg
5.		;		mm Hg
6.		;		mm Hg
7.		;		mm Hg

Suspected abnormality: Hypotension with nitroprusside therapy

Comments: The contour of this arterial pressure is somewhat unusual as a result of the tachycardia, which shortens the duration of diastolic runoff, and the induced vasodilatation, which increases stroke volume (by decreasing resistance) and facilitates rapid runoff peripherally.

Patient profile 4

A 49-year-old woman with a history of cardiomyopathy was admitted to the CCU with clinical symptoms of pulmonary edema despite medical management for congestive failure. Invasive hemodynamic assessment revealed a cardiac index of 2.0 L/min/m^2 and the following eight pressure tracings (pp. 135 to 142).

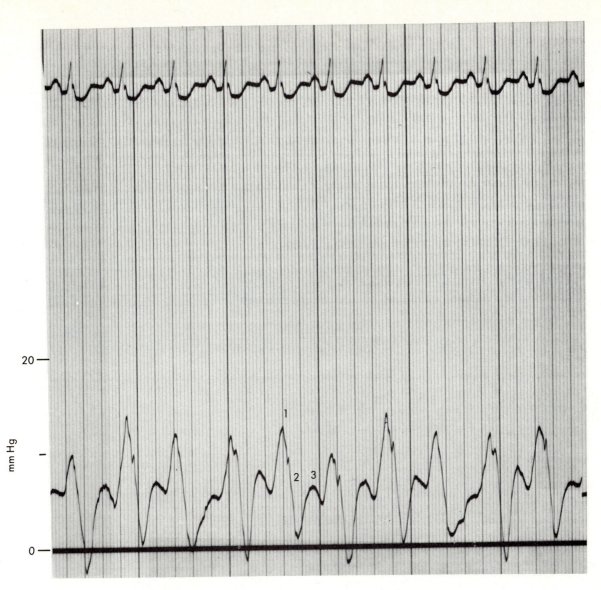

ANALYSIS

Rhythm: Sinus tachycardia

Pressure(s): RA

Waveform characteristics and measurements:

1.	*a* Wave	;	15 mm Hg
2.	*x* Descent	;	mm Hg
3.	*v* Wave	;	7 mm Hg
4.		;	mm Hg
5.		;	mm Hg
6.		;	mm Hg
7.		;	mm Hg

Suspected abnormality: RV failure

Comments: The *a* wave is prominent and elevated (15 mm Hg), indicating an increased resistance to RV filling. In this case the cause is long-standing left-sided heart failure.

135

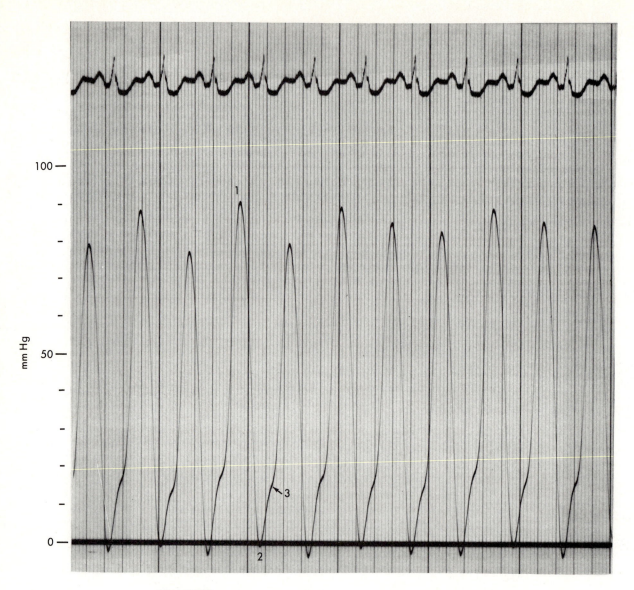

ANALYSIS

Rhythm: Sinus tachycardia

Pressure(s): RV

Waveform characteristics and measurements:

1.	RV systolic	;	82	mm Hg
2.	Early diastolic dip	;	0	mm Hg
3.	RVedp	;	16	mm Hg
4.		;		mm Hg
5.		;		mm Hg
6.		;		mm Hg
7.		;		mm Hg

Suspected abnormality: RV failure

Comments: Note the similarity between the measured RVedp and the *a* wave of the previous RA pressure tracing (p. 135).

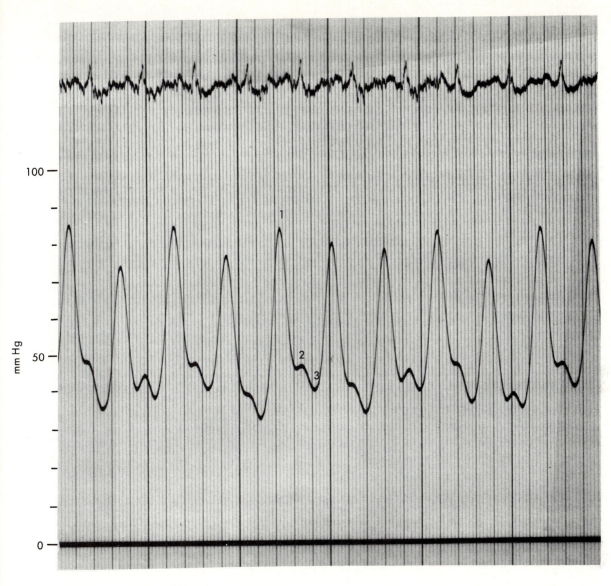

ANALYSIS

Rhythm: Sinus tachycardia

Pressure(s): PA

Waveform characteristics and measurements:

1.	PA systolic	;	80	mm Hg
2.	Dicrotic notch	;		mm Hg
3.	PA end-diastolic	;	38	mm Hg
4.		;		mm Hg
5.		;		mm Hg
6.		;		mm Hg
7.		;		mm Hg

Suspected abnormality: Acute pulmonary edema, 2^0 LV failure

Comments: Note the respiratory changes in this PA waveform, indicating a rapid respiratory rate usually seen in pulmonary edema.

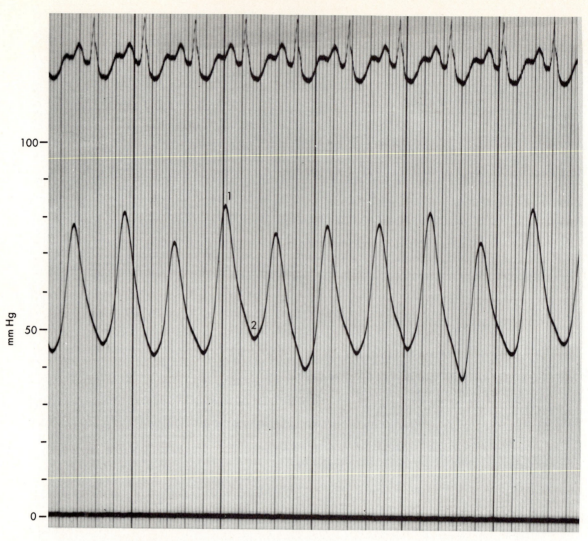

ANALYSIS

Rhythm: Sinus tachycardia

Pressure(s): PA

Waveform characteristics and measurements:

1.	PA systolic	;	75	mm Hg
2.	PA end-diastolic	;	45	mm Hg
3.		;		mm Hg
4.		;		mm Hg
5.		;		mm Hg
6.		;		mm Hg
7.		;		mm Hg

Suspected abnormality: Acute pulmonary edema, 2^0 LV failure

Comments: This is a slightly damped PA pressure waveform, as indicated by the rounded appearance and lack of dicrotic notch. Comparison with the previous PA pressure waveform (p. 137) reveals a slight reduction in pulse pressure. This is probably due to distal location of the catheter tip, which could be corrected by slight withdrawal of the Swan-Ganz catheter.

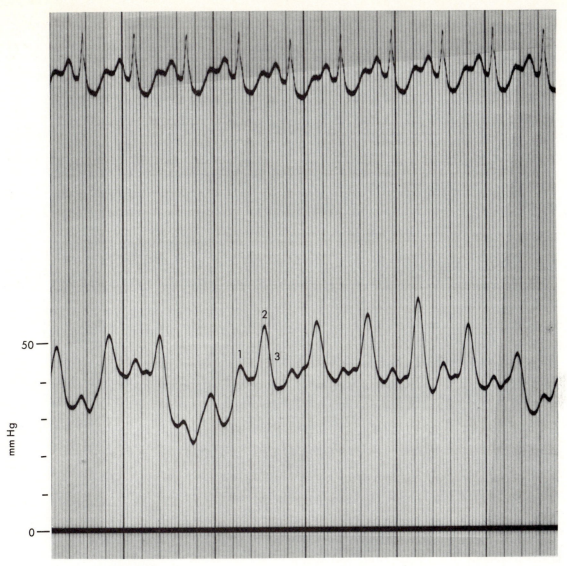

ANALYSIS

Rhythm: Sinus tachycardia

Pressure(s): PAW

Waveform characteristics and measurements:

1.	*a* Wave	;	40	mm Hg
2.	v Wave	;	52	mm Hg
3.	*y* Descent	;		mm Hg
4.	Mean	;	43	mm Hg
5.		;		mm Hg
6.		;		mm Hg
7.		;		mm Hg

Suspected abnormality: Acute pulmonary edema with mild mitral regurgitation, 2^0 LV failure

Comments: Note the dominant *v* wave indicative of mitral regurgitation, probably functional, secondary to LV failure.

139

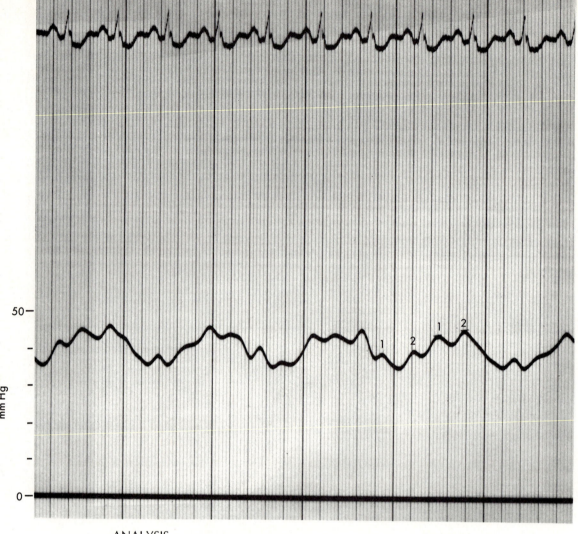

ANALYSIS

Rhythm: Sinus tachycardia

Pressure(s): PAW

Waveform characteristics and measurements:

1.	*a* Wave	;	41	mm Hg
2.	*v* Wave	;	41	mm Hg
3.	Mean	;	39	mm Hg
4.		;		mm Hg
5.		;		mm Hg
6.		;		mm Hg
7.		;		mm Hg

Suspected abnormality: Acute pulmonary edema

Comments: Comparison of this PAW waveform with the previous PAW (p. 139) emphasizes the damped quality of this waveform, probably due to a clot at the tip of the catheter. Deflation of the balloon, aspiration, and gentle flushing while in the PA position are necessary to obtain an accurate PAW pressure waveform.

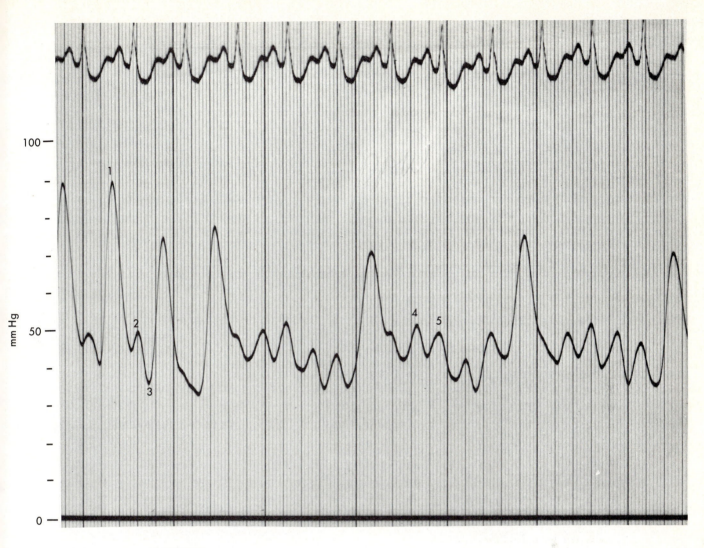

ANALYSIS

Rhythm: Sinus tachycardia

Pressure(s): PA/PAW

Waveform characteristics and measurements:

1.	PA systolic	;	85	mm Hg
2.	Dicrotic notch	;		mm Hg
3.	PA end-diastolic	;	38	mm Hg
4.	PAW *v* wave	;	48	mm Hg
5.	PAW *a* wave	;	49	mm Hg
6.		;		mm Hg
7.		;		mm Hg

Suspected abnormality: Acute pulmonary edema

Comments: The first two beats are clearly a PA pressure. The following waveforms are mixed PA/PAW due to forward migration of the catheter tip. The pressure change from PA to PAW appears to be cyclical and regular, indicating that the changes follow the respiratory pattern. Slight withdrawal of the catheter tip should eliminate this problem.

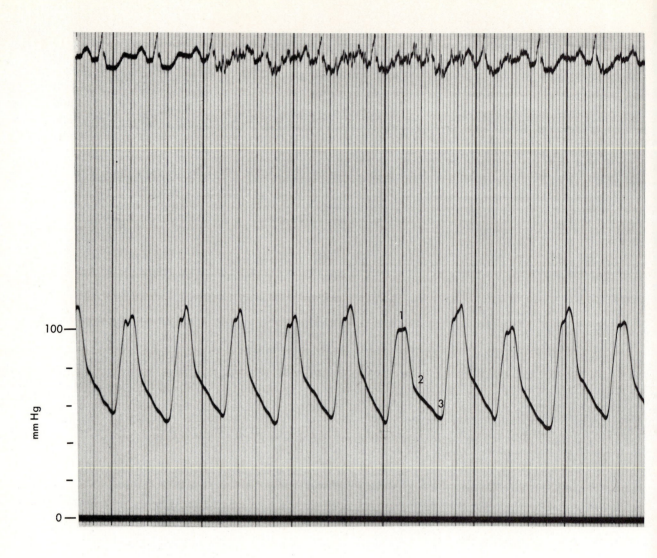

ANALYSIS

Rhythm: Sinus tachycardia

Pressure(s): Radial artery

Waveform characteristics and measurements:

1.	Arterial systolic	;	100	mm Hg
2.	Dicrotic notch	;		mm Hg
3.	Arterial diastolic	;	55	mm Hg
4.		;		mm Hg
5.		;		mm Hg
6.		;		mm Hg
7.		;		mm Hg

Suspected abnormality: Mild hypotension

Comments:

Patient profile 5

A 27-year-old woman was admitted to the CCU with marked hypotension and increasing symptoms of both right- and left-sided heart failure, including dyspnea, ascites, and cyanosis. Past medical history included a myomectomy and mitral valve replacement 6 years previously for IHSS. A temporary demand pacemaker was inserted, and hemodynamic instrumentation was initiated. The patient's cardiac index was 1.2 L/min/m^2, and the following seven hemodynamic pressures (pp. 144 to 150) were obtained.

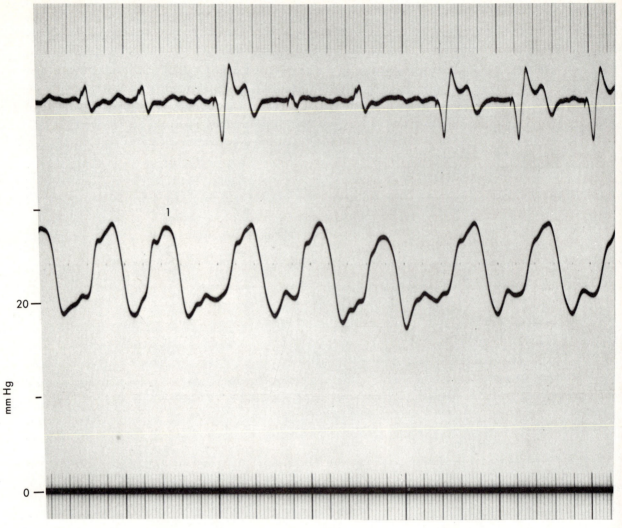

mm Hg

20 —

0 —

ANALYSIS

Rhythm: Atrial fibrillation with temporary demand pacemaker at 70 BPM

Pressure(s): RA

Waveform characteristics and measurements:

1.	*v* Wave ;	30 mm Hg
2.	;	mm Hg
3.	;	mm Hg
4.	;	mm Hg
5.	;	mm Hg
6.	;	mm Hg
7.	;	mm Hg

Suspected abnormality: Severe tricuspid regurgitation

Comments: The presence of atrial fibrillation accounts for the lack of an *a* wave in this RA pressure waveform. The elevated *v* wave of 30 mm Hg is caused by regurgitation of blood into the RA during RV systole. This is probably functional tricuspid regurgitation secondary to a dilated right ventricle.

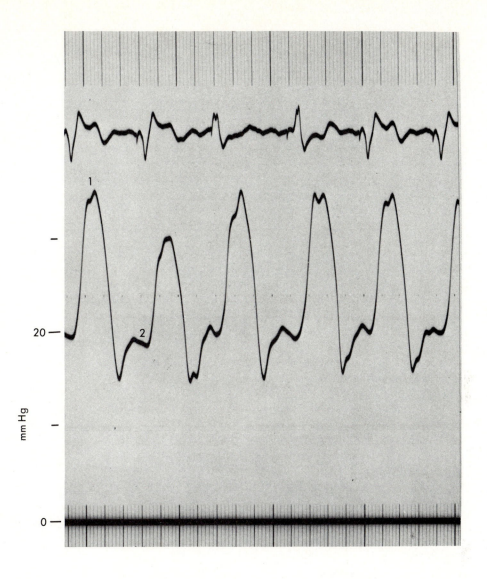

ANALYSIS

Rhythm: Atrial fibrillation with temporary demand pacemaker at 70 BPM

Pressure(s): RV

Waveform characteristics and measurements:

1.	RV systolic	;	35	mm Hg
2.	RV diastolic dip	;		mm Hg
3.	RV end-diastolic	;	20	mm Hg
4.		;		mm Hg
5.		;		mm Hg
6.		;		mm Hg
7.		;		mm Hg

Suspected abnormality: RV failure

Comments: The RV systolic pressure is only mildly elevated (35 mm Hg), but the RV end-diastolic pressure of 20 mm Hg is indicative of severe RV failure.

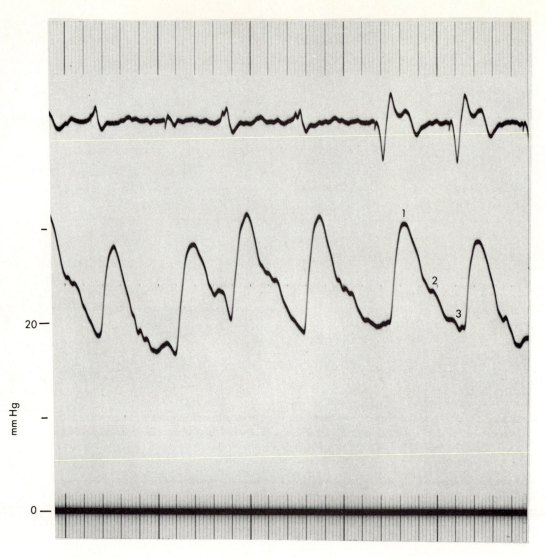

ANALYSIS

Rhythm: Atrial fibrillation with temporary demand pacemaker at 70 BPM

Pressure(s): PA

Waveform characteristics and measurements:

1.	PA systolic	;	32	mm Hg
2.	Dicrotic notch	;		mm Hg
3.	PA end-diastolic	;	20	mm Hg
4.		;		mm Hg
5.		;		mm Hg
6.		;		mm Hg
7.		;		mm Hg

Suspected abnormality: LV failure

Comments: The PA systolic pressure is only mildly elevated, possibly due to diminished forward blood flow from the RV. The end-diastolic pressure of 20 mm Hg is moderately elevated, indicating LV failure.

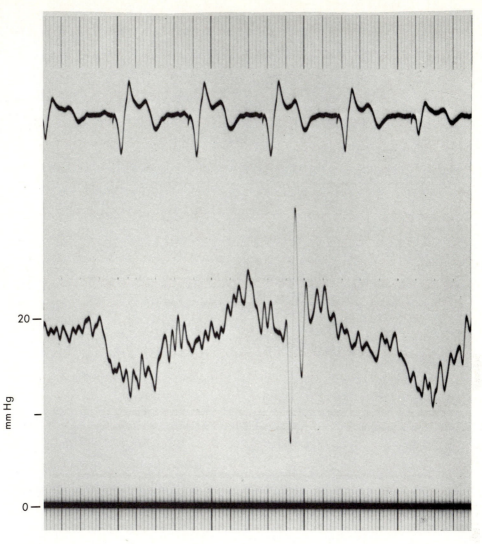

ANALYSIS

Rhythm: Paced at 70 BPM

Pressure(s): PAW

Waveform characteristics and measurements:

1.	Mean	;	17	mm Hg
2.		;		mm Hg
3.		;		mm Hg
4.		;		mm Hg
5.		;		mm Hg
6.		;		mm Hg
7.		;		mm Hg

Suspected abnormality: LV failure

Comments: This PAW pressure waveform appears to have much noise or interference, making accurate interpretation difficult. Minimizing the length of pressure tubing may correct this problem. The elevated mean pressure of 17 mm Hg indicates mild LV failure.

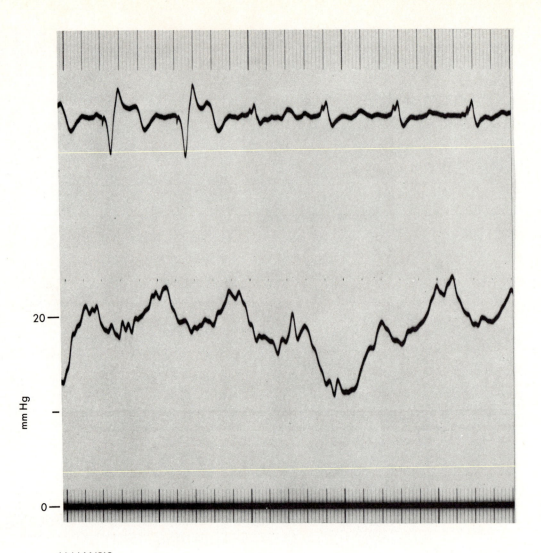

ANALYSIS

Rhythm: Atrial fibrillation with temporary demand pacemaker at 70 BPM

Pressure(s): PAW

Waveform characteristics and measurements:

1.	_v_ Wave	;	22 mm Hg
2.	Mean	;	20 mm Hg
3.		;	mm Hg
4.		;	mm Hg
5.		;	mm Hg
6.		;	mm Hg
7.		;	mm Hg

Suspected abnormality: LV failure

Comments: The _a_ wave is absent in this PAW pressure waveform due to atrial fibrillation. The elevated mean pressure of 20 mm Hg suggests LV failure. The
contour of this PAW waveform is improved in comparison with that on
p. 147.

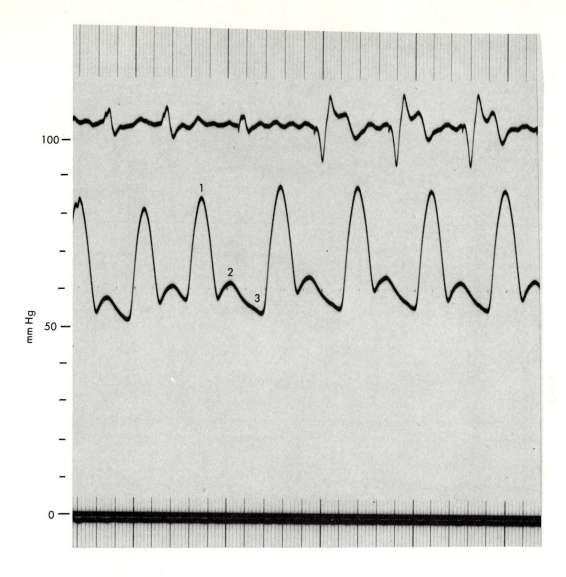

ANALYSIS

Rhythm: Atrial fibrillation/atrial flutter with demand pacemaker at 70 BPM

Pressure(s): Radial artery

Waveform characteristics and measurements:

1.	Arterial systolic	;	84 mm Hg
2.	Dicrotic notch	;	mm Hg
3.	Arterial end-diastolic	;	57 mm Hg
4.		;	mm Hg
5.		;	mm Hg
6.		;	mm Hg
7.		;	mm Hg

Suspected abnormality: Hypotension

Comments: This low arterial pressure with narrow pulse pressure (27 mm Hg) is due to a small stroke volume.

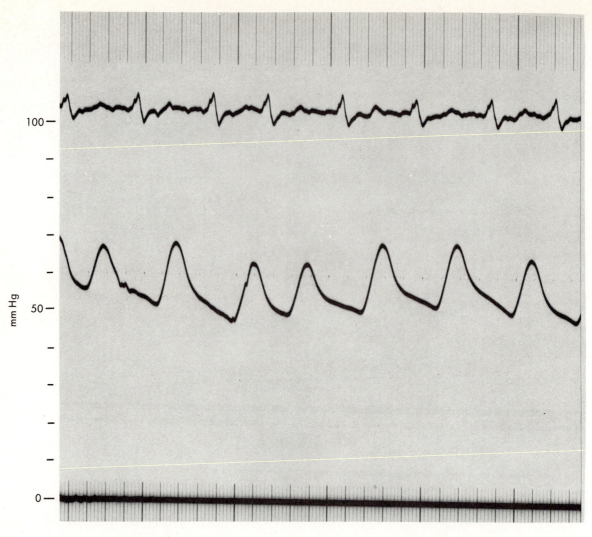

ANALYSIS

Rhythm: Atrial fibrillation

Pressure(s): Radial artery

Waveform characteristics and measurements:

1.	Arterial systolic	;	68 mm Hg
2.	Arterial end-diastolic	;	52 mm Hg
3.		;	mm Hg
4.		;	mm Hg
5.		;	mm Hg
6.		;	mm Hg
7.		;	mm Hg

Suspected abnormality: Damped arterial pressure

Comments: Comparison of this pressure with the arterial pressure waveform on p. 149 shows a pressure of much lower value with a narrower pulse pressure. Additionally, the contour has a rounded appearance, a slow upstroke, and poorly defined dicrotic notch. This could be due to a clot at the tip of the catheter or lodging of the catheter tip against the wall of the artery. Catheter manipulation or aspiration and flushing may be required to improve this pressure waveform.

Patient profile 6

A 41-year-old woman with the confirmed diagnosis of cardiomyopathy and progressive heart failure was admitted for evaluation of possible cardiac transplantation. Hemodynamic instrumentation was performed to assess the patient's response to vasodilator therapy. Hemodynamic data obtained were a cardiac index of 2.2 L/min/m^2 and the following six pressure tracings (pp. 152 to 157).

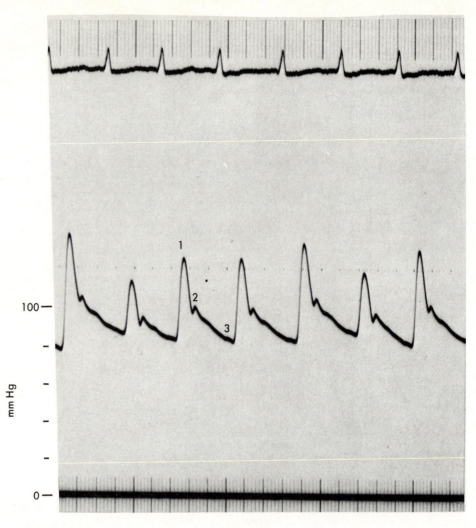

ANALYSIS

Rhythm: Atrial fibrillation

Pressure(s): Radial artery

Waveform characteristics and measurements:

1.	Arterial systolic	;	132	mm Hg
2.	Dicrotic notch	;		mm Hg
3.	Arterial diastolic	;	80	mm Hg
4.		;		mm Hg
5.		;		mm Hg
6.		;		mm Hg
7.		;		mm Hg

Suspected abnormality: Normal

Comments: Note the beat-to-beat variation in arterial pressure, reflecting changes in stroke volume, as a result of changes in filling time of the LV. The shorter the RR interval, the shorter the diastolic filling period and hence the lesser stroke volume. Compensatory vasoconstriction, which increases afterload, is responsible for maintaining this blood pressure within normal levels.

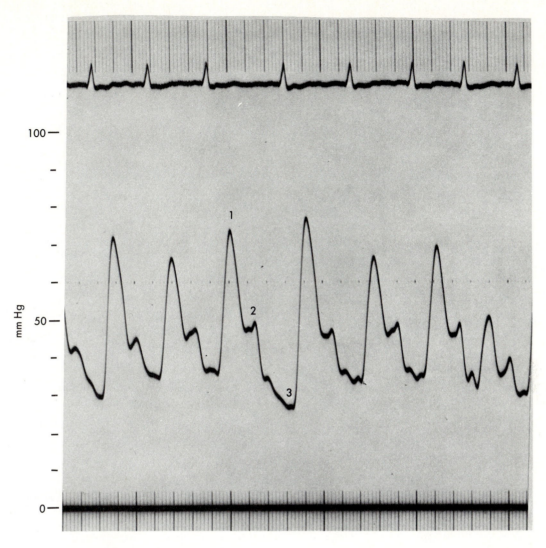

ANALYSIS

Rhythm: Atrial fibrillation

Pressure(s): PA

1.	PA systolic	;	62	mm Hg
2.	Dicrotic notch	;		mm Hg
3.	PA end-diastolic	;	30	mm Hg
4.		;		mm Hg
5.		;		mm Hg
6.		;		mm Hg
7.		;		mm Hg

Suspected abnormality: Pulmonary hypertension secondary to LV failure and mitral regurgitation

Comments: Note the extra notch on the dicrotic notch. This may represent retrograde transmission of an elevated *v* wave from the LA pressure due to mitral regurgitation. There is a more pronounced phase delay of this systolic event due to the retrograde transmission of the pressure. The elevated PAedp of 30 mm Hg indicates LV failure.

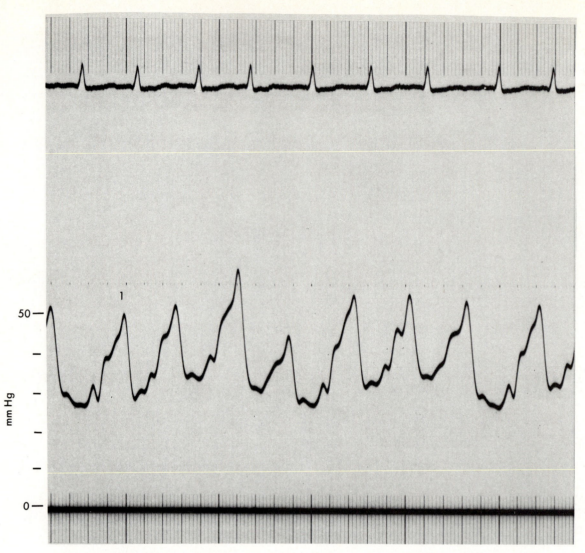

ANALYSIS

Rhythm: Atrial fibrillation

Pressure(s): PAW

Waveform characteristics and measurements:

1. _____ *v* Wave _____ ; _____ 47 _____ mm Hg

2. _____ ; _____ mm Hg

3. _____ ; _____ mm Hg

4. _____ ; _____ mm Hg

5. _____ ; _____ mm Hg

6. _____ ; _____ mm Hg

7. _____ ; _____ mm Hg

Suspected abnormality: Mitral regurgitation with CHF

Comments: The loss of electrical atrial depolarization in atrial fibrillation results in a loss of mechanical atrial systole, and therefore no *a* waves are evident in the PAW pressure waveform. The numerous small waves preceding the *v* waves are probably fibrillatory waves. The elevated *v* wave of 47 mm Hg is due to mitral regurgitation, probably functional.

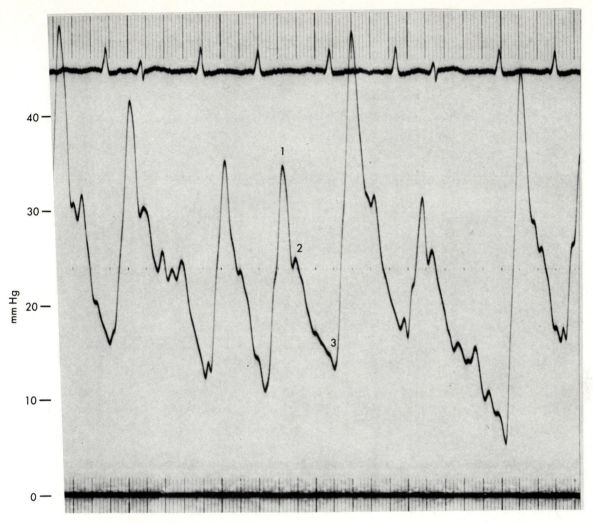

ANALYSIS

Rhythm: Atrial fibrillation

Pressure(s): PA

Waveform characteristics and measurements:

1.	PA systolic	;	40	mm Hg
2.	Dicrotic notch	;		mm Hg
3.	PA end-diastolic	;	15	mm Hg
4.		;		mm Hg
5.		;		mm Hg
6.		;		mm Hg
7.		;		mm Hg

Suspected abnormality: Mild pulmonary hypertension during afterload reduction

Comments: This PA pressure tracing is on a scale different from that of the PA pressure tracing on p. 153, thus altering the overall contour. The values of this PA pressure are lower, however, because of nitroprusside administration. The PAedp is markedly reduced (from 30 to 15 mm Hg), indicating a decrease in LV preload due to enhanced forward output and venous pooling as a result of nitroprusside.

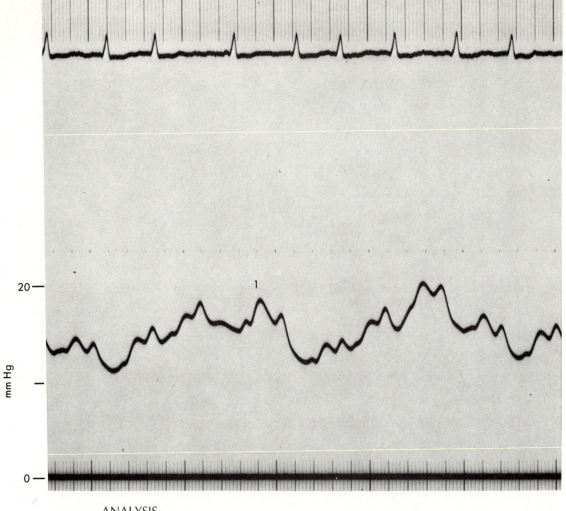

ANALYSIS

Rhythm: Atrial fibrillation

Pressure(s): PAW

Waveform characteristics and measurements:

1.	*v* Wave	;	18	mm Hg
2.	Mean	;	16	mm Hg
3.		;		mm Hg
4.		;		mm Hg
5.		;		mm Hg
6.		;		mm Hg
7.		;		mm Hg

Suspected abnormality: Improved PAW pressure during afterload reduction

Comments: This PAW pressure tracing is also recorded on a scale different from that of the previous PAW pressure (p. 154). The *v* wave, however, is markedly reduced (from 47 to 18 mm Hg) because of nitroprusside therapy. This is due to afterload reduction, which has facilitated and enhanced forward blood flow and reduced retrograde blood flow into the left atrium. The mean pressure of 16 mm Hg indicates only mild CHF.

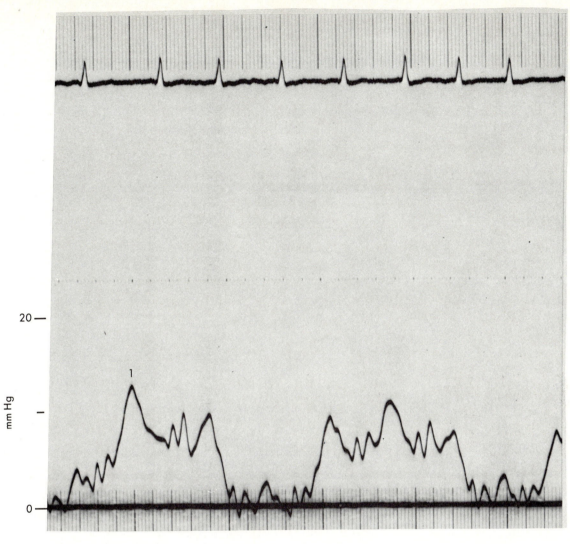

ANALYSIS

Rhythm: Atrial fibrillation

Pressure(s): PAW

Waveform characteristics and measurements:

1.	*v* Wave	;	8	mm Hg
2.	Mean	;	7	mm Hg
3.		;		mm Hg
4.		;		mm Hg
5.		;		mm Hg
6.		;		mm Hg
7.		;		mm Hg

Suspected abnormality: (?) Relative hypovolemia secondary to afterload reduction

Comments: The further decrease in PAW pressure with nitroprusside administration may reflect a state of relative hypovolemia secondary to venodilatation and venous pooling. If there are concomitant signs of hypoperfusion, this low PAW pressure of 7 mm Hg might indicate the need for volume administration.

Patient profile 7

A 73-year-old man was admitted to the CCU because of the increased occurrence of syncopal episodes and the presence of complete heart block. Because of the clinical suspicion of CHF, hemodynamic monitoring was initiated. The following four pressure tracings (pp. 159 to 162) disclose the hemodynamic data obtained and their correlation to the cardiac rhythm.

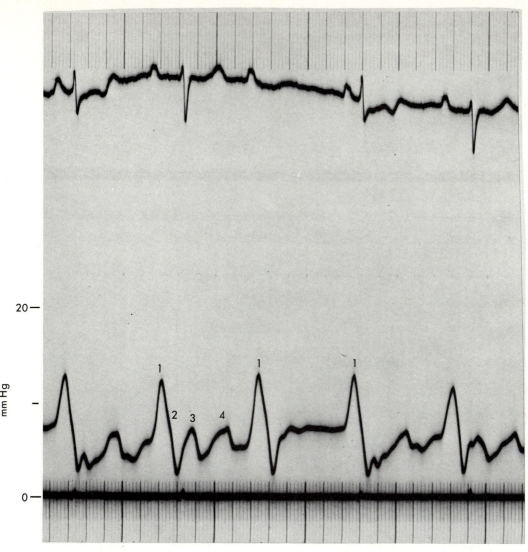

ANALYSIS

Rhythm: Second-degree AV block with Wenckebach phenomenon

Pressure(s): RA

Waveform characteristics and measurements:

1.	*a* Wave	;	12	mm Hg
2.	*x* Descent	;		mm Hg
3.	*c* Wave	;		mm Hg
4.	*v* Wave	;	7	mm Hg
5.	Mean	;	9	mm Hg
6.		;		mm Hg
7.		;		mm Hg

Suspected abnormality: Mild right-sided heart failure

Comments: Note the minimal time delay between the electrical and mechanical events, suggesting use of a miniature transducer connected directly to the catheter without the use of any extension tubing. The RA *a* wave of 12 mm Hg suggests some resistance to RV filling, as in mild RV failure. Note also the third RA *a* wave corresponding to the preceding P wave of the ECG. The conduction is blocked, however, so ventricular depolarization does not occur and therefore there is no succeeding *v* wave.

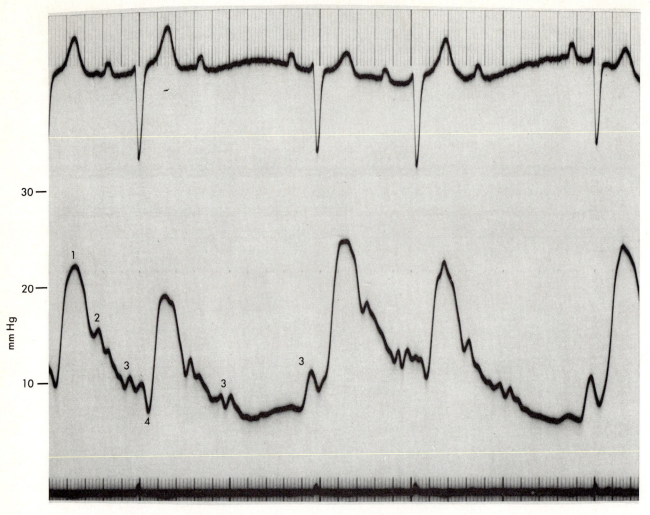

ANALYSIS

Rhythm: Second-degree AV block with Wenckebach phenomenon

Pressure(s): PA

Waveform characteristics and measurements:

1.	PA systolic	;	25	mm Hg
2.	Dicrotic notch	;		mm Hg
3.	*a* Wave	;	12	mm Hg
4.	PA end-diastolic	;	13	mm Hg
5.		;		mm Hg
6.		;		mm Hg
7.		;		mm Hg

Suspected abnormality: Normal

Comments: Note the retrograde transmission of the LA *a* wave in this PA pressure waveform and its correlation with the P wave of the ECG. Note also the increase in the PA systolic pressure following the nonconducted P wave. This is due to increase in ejection because of the increased duration of ventricular filling.

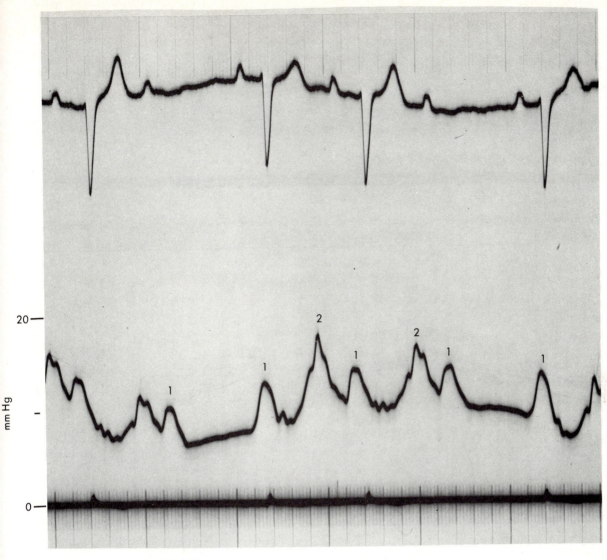

ANALYSIS

Rhythm: Second-degree AV block with Wenckebach phenomenon

Pressure(s): PAW

Waveform characteristics and measurements:

1.	*a* Wave	;	14 mm Hg
2.	*v* Wave	;	16 mm Hg
3.	Mean	;	12 mm Hg
4.		;	mm Hg
5.		;	mm Hg
6.		;	mm Hg
7.		;	mm Hg

Suspected abnormality: Mild CHF

Comments: Each atrial depolarization (P wave) is followed by atrial systole (PAW *a* wave). However, since every third impulse is not conducted, a *v* wave does not follow each *a* wave. Careful analysis of this tracing shows PAW *a* waves following each ECG P wave and a *v* wave after each ventricular depolarization, albeit at a different rate.

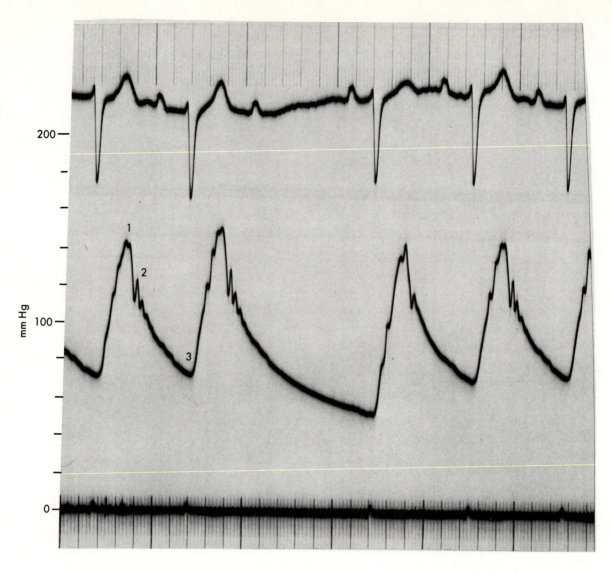

ANALYSIS

Rhythm: Second-degree AV block with Wenckebach phenomenon

Pressure(s): Radial artery

Waveform characteristics and measurements:

1.	Arterial systolic	;	143	mm Hg
2.	Dicrotic notch	;		mm Hg
3.	Arterial diastolic	;	70	mm Hg
4.		;		mm Hg
5.		;		mm Hg
6.		;		mm Hg
7.		;		mm Hg

Suspected abnormality: Normal

Comments: Note the lack of conduction of the third impulse, causing a pause in the arterial pulse and extending the diastolic period of the previous waveform.

Patient profile 8

A 71-year-old man was admitted to the ICU following aortic valve replacement and coronary artery bypass graft to the LAD. A Swan-Ganz catheter, a radial artery catheter, and a temporary pacemaker wire were placed at the time of surgery. He subsequently developed complete heart block, and the pacemaker was turned on at a rate of 70 BPM. The following three hemodynamic pressure waveforms (pp. 164 to 166) were obtained.

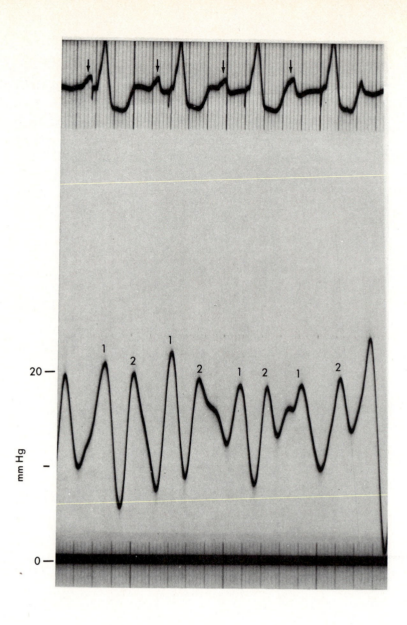

ANALYSIS

Rhythm: Paced at 70 BPM (Note pacemaker spikes and P waves in ECG.)

Pressure(s): RA

Waveform characteristics and measurements:

1.	*a* Waves	; 20	mm Hg
2.	*v* Waves	; 20	mm Hg
3.	Mean	; 15	mm Hg
4.		;	mm Hg
5.		;	mm Hg
6.		;	mm Hg
7.		;	mm Hg

Suspected abnormality: Hypervolemia or RV failure

Comments: Note the RA *a* waves corresponding to the appearance of P waves in the ECG. Note also the prominent *a* and *v* waves with rapid *x* and *y* descent, which may be due to a noncompliant RA and RV.

164

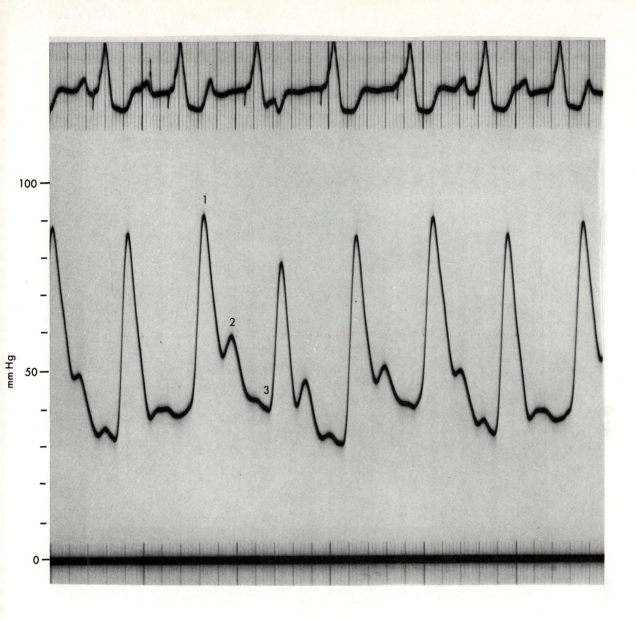

ANALYSIS

Rhythm: Paced at 70 BPM (Note pacemaker spikes and P waves in ECG.)

Pressure(s): PA

Waveform characteristics and measurements:

1.	PA systolic	;	85	mm Hg
2.	Dicrotic notch	;		mm Hg
3.	PA end-diastolic	;	35	mm Hg
4.		;		mm Hg
5.		;		mm Hg
6.		;		mm Hg
7.		;		mm Hg

Suspected abnormality: Hypervolemia

Comments:

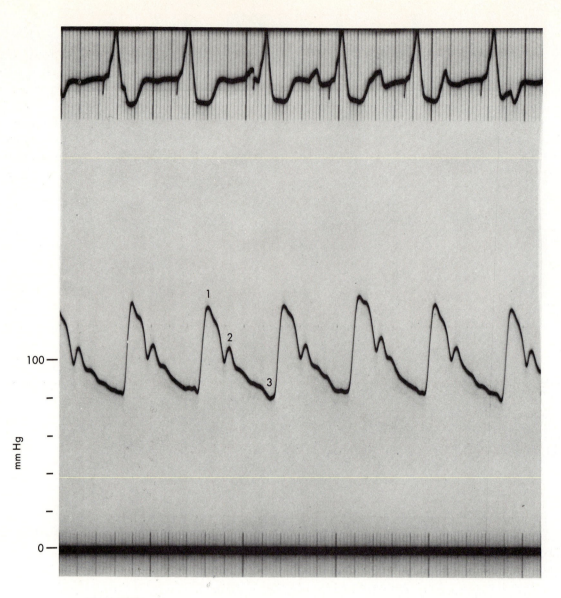

ANALYSIS

Rhythm: Paced at 70 BPM (Note pacemaker spikes and P waves appearing in ECG.)

Pressure(s): Radial artery

Waveform characteristics and measurements:

1.	Arterial systolic	;	112 mm Hg
2.	Dicrotic notch	;	mm Hg
3.	Arterial diastolic	;	90 mm Hg
4.		;	mm Hg
5.		;	mm Hg
6.		;	mm Hg
7.		;	mm Hg

Suspected abnormality: Normal

Comments:

Patient profile 9

A 30-year-old man was admitted to the CCU with complaints of dyspnea on exertion and the occurrence of blackout spells. Prior cardiac catheterization confirmed the diagnosis of severe primary pulmonary hypertension. Hemodynamic instrumentation was instituted to evaluate his hemodynamic response to a trial of vasodilator therapy in an attempt to control his pulmonary hypertension. Unfortunately, as the next seven pressure tracings (pp. 168 to 174) illustrate, this patient's pulmonary hypertension was very severe and resistant to vasodilator therapy, including nitroprusside and isoproterenol, making him a candidate for the heart-lung transplant program.

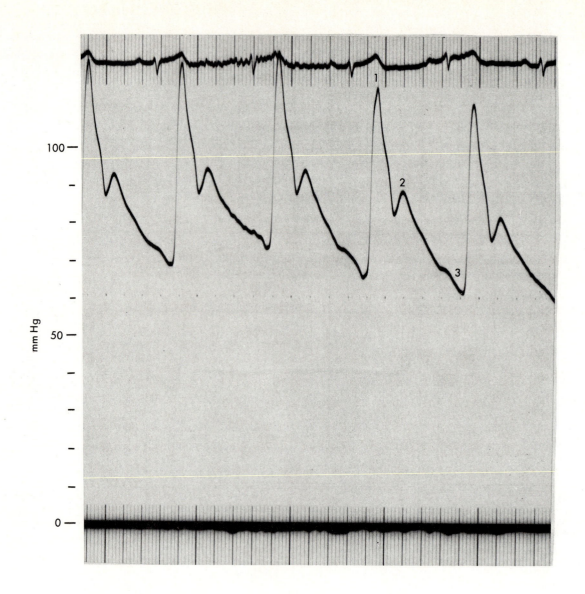

ANALYSIS

Rhythm: NSR

Pressure(s): PA

Waveform characteristics and measurements:

1.	PA systolic	;	119	mm Hg
2.	Dicrotic notch	;		mm Hg
3.	PA end-diastolic	;	70	mm Hg
4.		;		mm Hg
5.		;		mm Hg
6.		;		mm Hg
7.		;		mm Hg

Suspected abnormality: Severe pulmonary hypertension

Comments:

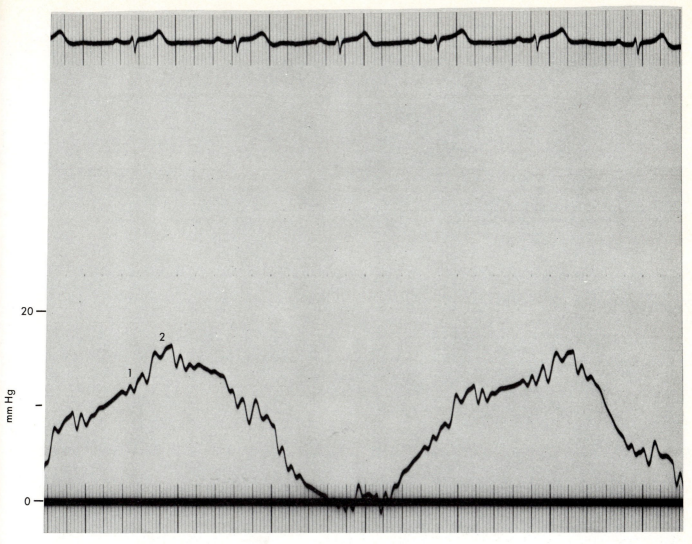

ANALYSIS

Rhythm: NSR

Pressure(s): PAW

Waveform characteristics and measurements:

1. _____ *a* Wave _____ ; _____ mm Hg

2. _____ *v* Wave _____ ; _____ mm Hg

3. _____ Mean _____ ; _____ 9 _____ mm Hg

4. _____ ; _____ mm Hg

5. _____ ; _____ mm Hg

6. _____ ; _____ mm Hg

7. _____ ; _____ mm Hg

Suspected abnormality: Normal

Comments: Exaggerated respiratory changes make exact identification of the *a* and *v* waves difficult. That exact an identification is not necessary, however, since neither the *a* nor the *v* wave is particularly dominant or elevated. In this case a mean PAW pressure, which averages the pressure changes during one complete respiratory cycle, more closely reflects the LVedp. The exaggerated respiratory changes are commonly seen in patients with pulmonary hypertension.

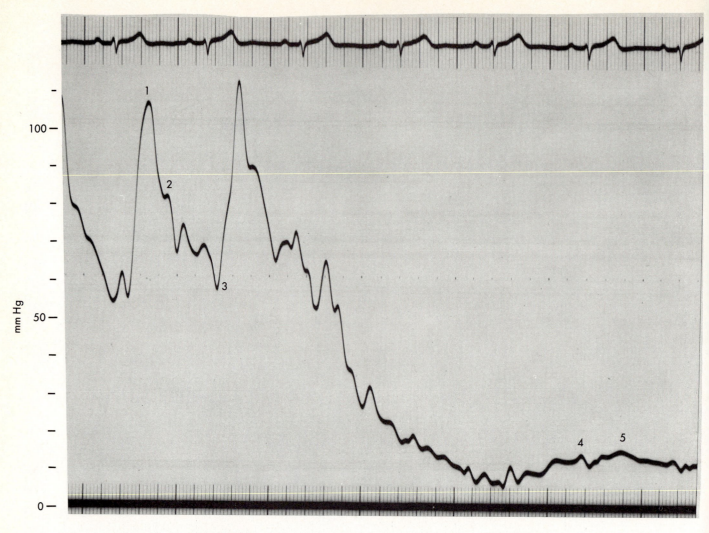

ANALYSIS

Rhythm: NSR

Pressure(s): PA to PAW

Waveform characteristics and measurements:

1.	PA systolic	;	108	mm Hg
2.	Dicrotic notch	;		mm Hg
3.	PA end-diastolic	;	55	mm Hg
4.	PAW *a* wave	;	10	mm Hg
5.	PAW *v* wave	;	10	mm Hg
6.		;		mm Hg
7.		;		mm Hg

Suspected abnormality: Severe primary pulmonary hypertension

Comments: The extremely high PA pressure (108/55) with normal PAW pressures reflects a high PVR due to pulmonary vascular disease. Heart failure can be ruled out as the cause in the presence of a normal PAW pressure of 10 mm Hg. In this case the PA pressure does not reflect the LVedp but, rather, the high PVR. Preload of the left ventricle can still be monitored, however, through measurement of the PAW pressure. This shows the importance of obtaining an initial correlation between the PAedp and PA pressures before using the PAedp to monitor the LVedp. In this case, only the PAW pressure can be used to monitor LV preload.

170

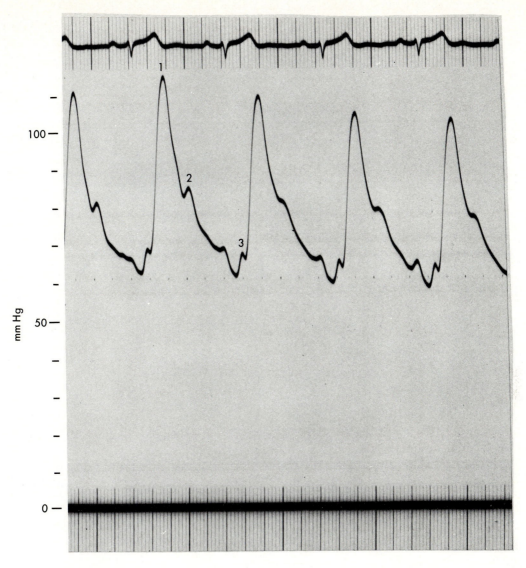

ANALYSIS

Rhythm: NSR

Pressure(s): PA

Waveform characteristics and measurements:

1.	PA systolic	;	110	mm Hg
2.	Dicrotic notch	;		mm Hg
3.	PA end-diastolic	;	60	mm Hg
4.		;		mm Hg
5.		;		mm Hg
6.		;		mm Hg
7.		;		mm Hg

Suspected abnormality: Severe primary pulmonary hypertension

Comments: This is the PA pressure following nitroprusside infusion of 133 μg/min for 20 minutes showing virtually no response to afterload reduction.

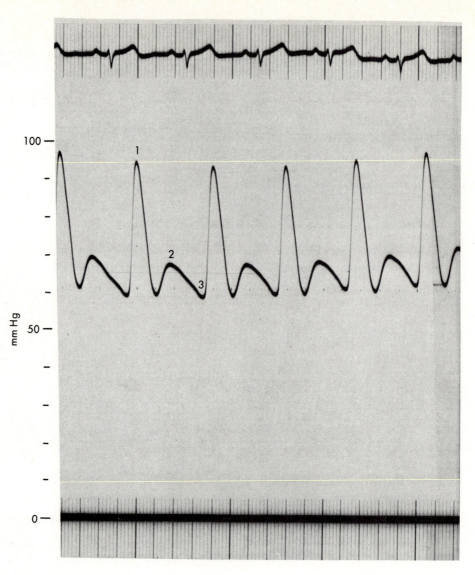

ANALYSIS

Rhythm: NSR

Pressure(s): Radial artery

Waveform characteristics and measurements:

1.	Arterial systolic	;	97	mm Hg
2.	Dicrotic notch	;		mm Hg
3.	Arterial diastolic	;	60	mm Hg
4.		;		mm Hg
5.		;		mm Hg
6.		;		mm Hg
7.		;		mm Hg

Suspected abnormality: Hypotension secondary to afterload reduction

Comments: This is the arterial pressure during nitroprusside therapy, reflecting a decrease in systolic pressure, enhanced, rapid ejection during systole, and rapid runoff during diastole.

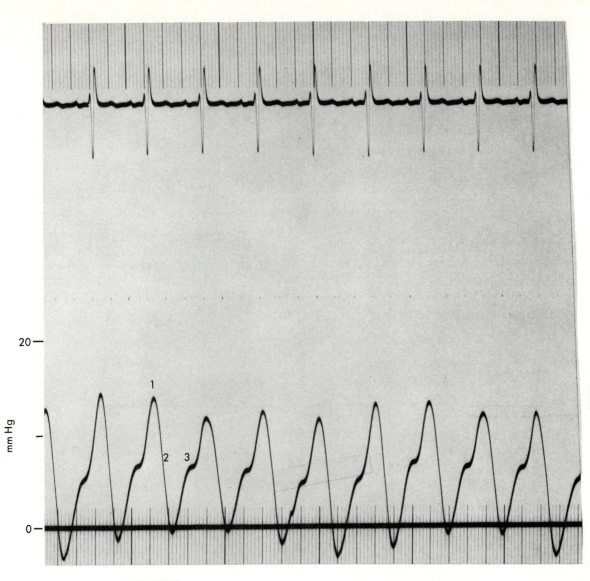

ANALYSIS

Rhythm: NSR (sensitivity increased)

Pressure(s): RA

Waveform characteristics and measurements:

1.	*a* Wave	;	12 mm Hg
2.	*x* Descent	;	mm Hg
3.	*v* Wave	;	7 mm Hg
4.	Mean	;	6 mm Hg
5.		;	mm Hg
6.		;	mm Hg
7.		;	mm Hg

Suspected abnormality: Normal

Comments: This RA pressure tracing was taken 24 hours after those on pp. 168 to 172 and shows a prominent *a* wave and *x* descent. This is probably due to hypertrophy of the RV secondary to pulmonary hypertension and high PVR.

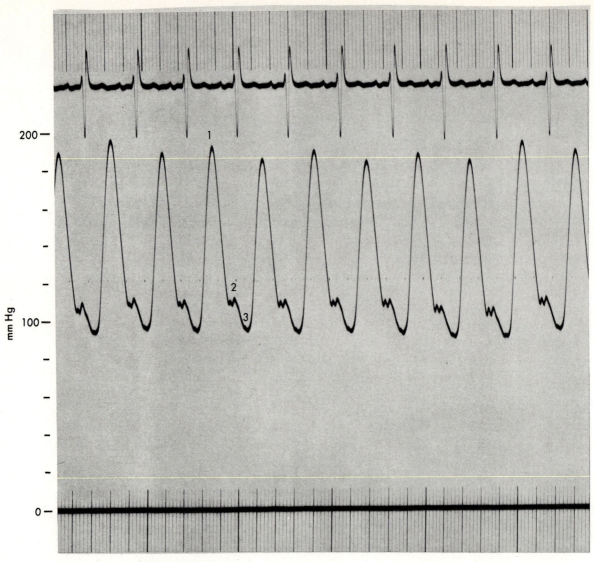

ANALYSIS

Rhythm: NSR (sensitivity increased)

Pressure(s): PA

Waveform characteristics and measurements:

1.	PA systolic	;	195	mm Hg
2.	Dicrotic notch	;		mm Hg
3.	PA end-diastolic	;	95	mm Hg
4.		;		mm Hg
5.		;		mm Hg
6.		;		mm Hg
7.		;		mm Hg

Suspected abnormality: Severe pulmonary hypertension unresponsive to isoproterenol infusion

Comments: This PA pressure tracing was obtained 24 hours after those on pp. 168 to 172 and during an infusion of isoproterenol in an attempt to reduce PVR and the PA pressure. Unfortunately the desired effect was not achieved, and the PA pressure rose even higher, resulting in immediate cessation of isoproterenol administration.

chapter 7

Self-assessment

This section consists of numerous and varied hemodynamic pressure tracings for the reader to assess his or her skill in identifying and interpreting both normal and abnormal pressure waveforms.

A systematic approach to identification of pressure waveforms is most useful. The following steps offer one method of waveform analysis. However, whatever method is used, consistently answering the following questions can minimize confusion.

1. What is the cardiac rhythm?

Knowledge of the patient's heart rhythm offers clues as to what to look for in the pressure waveform. With atrial fibrillation the atrial pressures (RA, LA, or PAW) will reveal only a *v* wave for each QRS complex. In AV dissociation it is possible to see unusually large cannon *a* waves in the atrial pressure waveform. The arterial pressure contour (either pulmonary artery or systemic artery), in atrial fibrillation, will exhibit marked variation in pulse pressure.

2. What type of waveform does it look like?

By this time, having seen numerous normal waveforms, you know what atrial pressures (RA, LA, and PAW), ventricular pressures, or arterial pressures look like. The answer to this question may be: "This pressure looks like what I know an atrial pressure looks like. I see a low pressure with an *a* wave and a *v* wave." Or it may be: "This looks like an arterial type of pressure with an upstroke, systole, dicrotic notch, and diastole." Or: "This pressure looks like a ventricular pressure with systolic pressure the same as the PA systolic pressure, but the diastolic pressure falling down to baseline."

3. Is the contour of the pressure waveform normal?

Having identified the pressure, it is important to note if the contour or the characteristics of the pressure waveform are normal. With the atrial pressure, is either the *a* or the *v* wave dominant? Is either the *x* or *y* descent prominent or abbreviated? With the arterial pressures (PA or arterial), is the upstroke rapid or slow? Is the dicrotic notch present or absent? Is the runoff period prolonged or abbreviated?

4. Is the value of the pressure waveform normal?

Having identified the pressure and assessed its characteristics, it is important to measure the value of the pressure and determine whether it falls within normal ranges. Look carefully at the value scale indicated on the left side of the tracing. With the atrial pressures (RA, LA, or PAW), a mean or average pressure is usually recorded. However, if the *v* wave is dominant and elevated, both the *a* and *v* waves should be measured and recorded. In the following tracings, you should indicate the values of both *a* and *v* waves. It is not necessary, however, to note the value of the *c* wave, even though you are asked to identify it. With the arterial pressure (PA and arterial), the systolic, diastolic, and mean values are recorded. It is not necessary to note the value of the dicrotic notch, only to identify its presence or absence.

A cautionary note regarding "normal values" must be mentioned here. The values of the hemodynamic pressures must always be correlated with the patient's clinical picture! For example, even though a mean PAW pressure of 8 mm Hg may be normal in one clinical setting, it may be abnormally low for the patient with a low cardiac output. No single hemodynamic parameter or measurement should be used to guide medical care.

5. What is the suspected abnormality?

Based on the answers to the four previous questions, it should be possible to reach some answer regarding possible abnormalities. Hemodynamic data can provide information regarding some cardiac abnormalities, but they are usually not used to provide actual diagnosis. This usually requires more extensive information obtained from echocardiography and cardiac catheterization.

In the following pressures you are asked to identify, there could be one or more pathologic conditions responsible for the pressure abnormalities. To avoid repetition, only the more likely abnormality is listed, although you may be correct in listing others.

One last word of caution before proceeding with the pressure waveform identification. Frequently there occur many small, regular and consistent pressure rises in hemodynamic pressure tracings. These pressure rises or oscillations are hemodynamically insignificant. Too often, having learned to identify the pressure characteristics of certain waveforms, there is a tendency to place emphasis on every little oscillation in the pressure waveform.

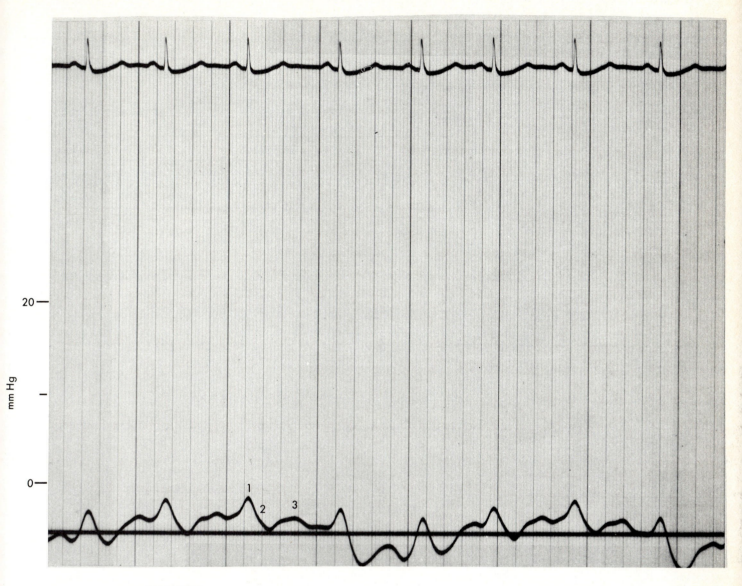

ANALYSIS

Rhythm:

Pressure(s):

Waveform characteristics and measurements:

1. _____ ; _____ mm Hg

2. _____ ; _____ mm Hg

3. _____ ; _____ mm Hg

4. _____ ; _____ mm Hg

5. _____ ; _____ mm Hg

6. _____ ; _____ mm Hg

7. _____ ; _____ mm Hg

Suspected abnormality:

Comments:

ANALYSIS

Rhythm: NSR

Pressure(s): RA

Waveform characteristics and measurements:

1. _____ *a* Wave _____ ; _____ 3 _____ mm Hg

2. _____ *x* Descent _____ ; _____ mm Hg

3. _____ *v* Wave _____ ; _____ 1 _____ mm Hg

4. _____ Mean _____ ; _____ 0-1 _____ mm Hg

5. _____ ; _____ mm Hg

6. _____ ; _____ mm Hg

7. _____ ; _____ mm Hg

Suspected abnormality: Hypovolemia or inaccurate placement of transducer air-reference level

Comments: The normal fall in RA pressure during inspiration becomes negative in this abnormally low RA pressure.

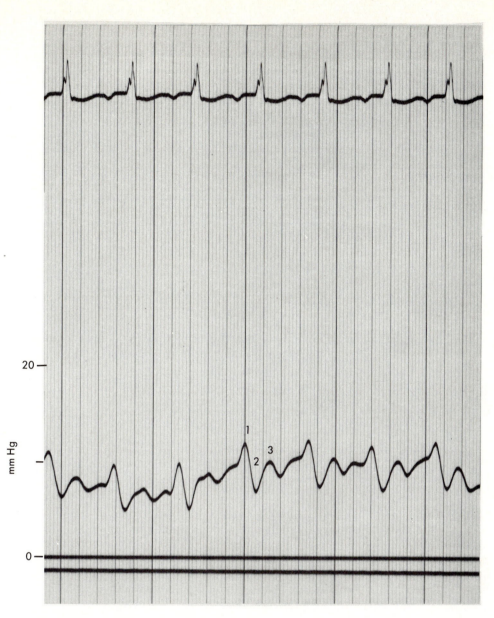

ANALYSIS

Rhythm:

Pressure(s):

Waveform characteristics and measurements:

1. _____ ; _____ mm Hg

2. _____ ; _____ mm Hg

3. _____ ; _____ mm Hg

4. _____ ; _____ mm Hg

5. _____ ; _____ mm Hg

6. _____ ; _____ mm Hg

7. _____ ; _____ mm Hg

Suspected abnormality:

Comments:

ANALYSIS

Rhythm: NSR

Pressure(s): PAW

Waveform characteristics and measurements:

1. _____ *a* Wave _____ ; _____ 11 _____ mm Hg

2. _____ *x* Descent _____ ; _____ mm Hg

3. _____ *v* Wave _____ ; _____ 9 _____ mm Hg

4. _____ Mean _____ ; _____ 10 _____ mm Hg

5. _____ ; _____ mm Hg

6. _____ ; _____ mm Hg

7. _____ ; _____ mm Hg

Suspected abnormality: Normal

Comments: Note the lack of delay between electrical and mechanical events suggesting use of a miniature transducer connected directly to the catheter hub.

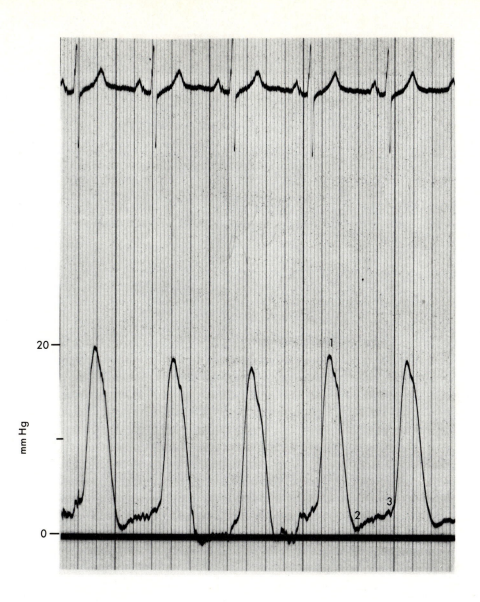

ANALYSIS

Rhythm:

Pressure(s):

Waveform characteristics and measurements:

1. _____ ; _____ mm Hg

2. _____ ; _____ mm Hg

3. _____ ; _____ mm Hg

4. _____ ; _____ mm Hg

5. _____ ; _____ mm Hg

6. _____ ; _____ mm Hg

7. _____ ; _____ mm Hg

Suspected abnormality:

Comments:

ANALYSIS

Rhythm: NSR

Pressure(s): RV

Waveform characteristics and measurements:

1.	RV systolic	; 19	mm Hg
2.	RV diastolic dip	; 0	mm Hg
3.	RV end-diastolic	; 3	mm Hg
4.		;	mm Hg
5.		;	mm Hg
6.		;	mm Hg
7.		;	mm Hg

Suspected abnormality: Normal

Comments:

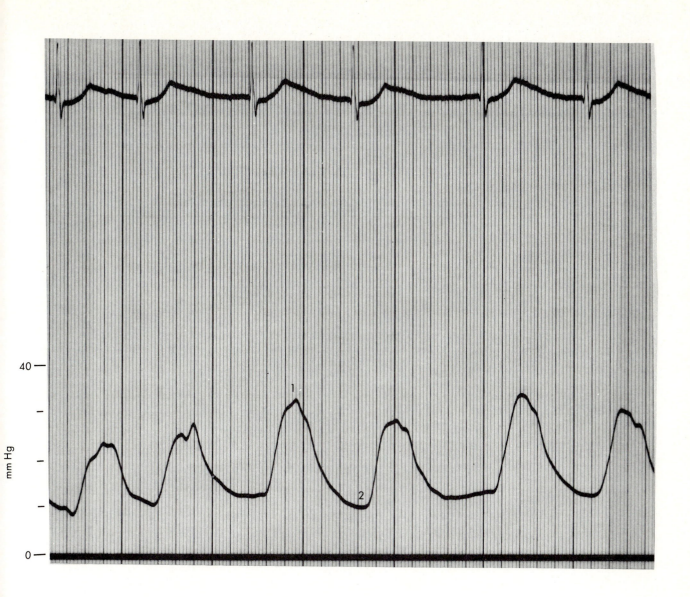

ANALYSIS

Rhythm:

Pressure(s):

Waveform characteristics and measurements:

1. _____ ; _____ mm Hg

2. _____ ; _____ mm Hg

3. _____ ; _____ mm Hg

4. _____ ; _____ mm Hg

5. _____ ; _____ mm Hg

6. _____ ; _____ mm Hg

7. _____ ; _____ mm Hg

Suspected abnormality:

Comments: **183**

ANALYSIS

Rhythm: Bradycardia (nodal escape?)

Pressure(s): PA

Waveform characteristics and measurements:

1.	PA systolic	;	28 mm Hg
2.	PA end-diastolic	;	11 mm Hg
3.		;	mm Hg
4.		;	mm Hg
5.		;	mm Hg
6.		;	mm Hg
7.		;	mm Hg

Suspected abnormality: Damped PA pressure

Comments: Note the rounded-out appearance of this PA pressure with a lack of distinct dicrotic notch. This is a damping effect from a clot at the tip of the catheter or an air bubble within the system.

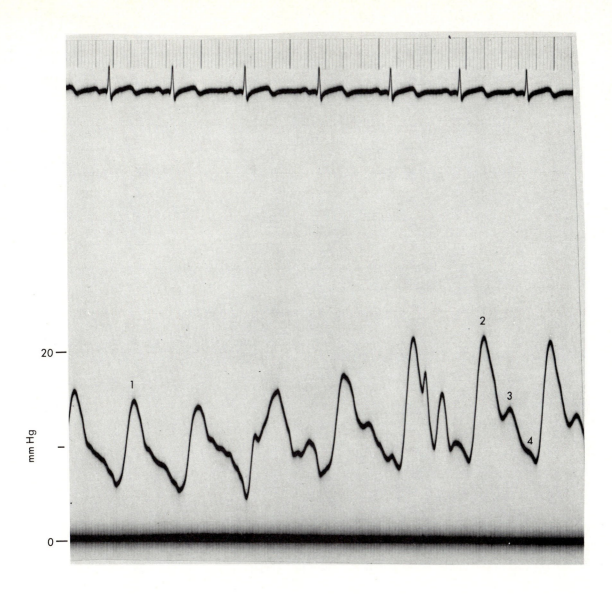

ANALYSIS

Rhythm:

Pressure(s):

Waveform characteristics and measurements:

1. _____ ; _____ mm Hg

2. _____ ; _____ mm Hg

3. _____ ; _____ mm Hg

4. _____ ; _____ mm Hg

5. _____ ; _____ mm Hg

6. _____ ; _____ mm Hg

7. _____ ; _____ mm Hg

Suspected abnormality:

Comments:

ANALYSIS

Rhythm: NSR

Pressure(s): PA

Waveform characteristics and measurements:

1.	Damped PA systolic	;	15	mm Hg
2.	PA systolic	;	20	mm Hg
3.	Dicrotic notch	;		mm Hg
4.	PA end-diastolic	;	8	mm Hg
5.		;		mm Hg
6.		;		mm Hg
7.		;		mm Hg

Suspected abnormality: Normal

Comments: The catheter tip was probably lodged against the wall of the pulmonary artery, causing a damped pressure contour. Slight movement of the catheter freed the catheter tip and improved the pressure tracing (note the last three waveforms).

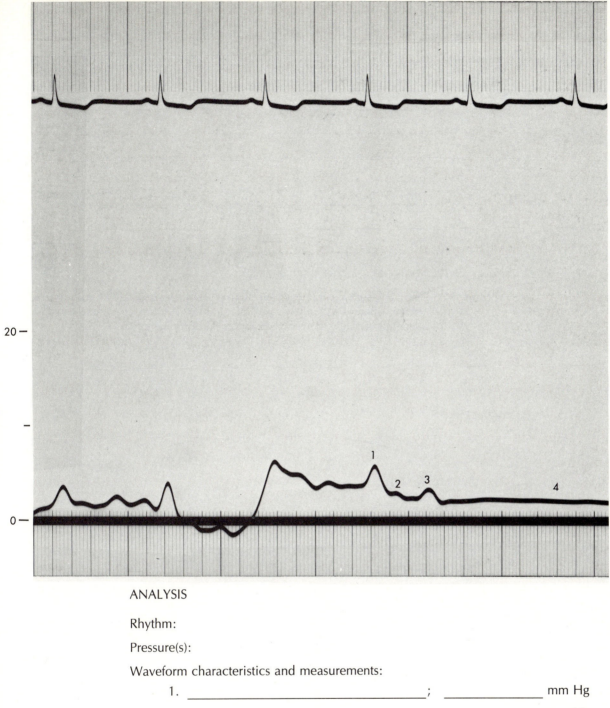

ANALYSIS

Rhythm:

Pressure(s):

Waveform characteristics and measurements:

1. _____ ; _____ mm Hg

2. _____ ; _____ mm Hg

3. _____ ; _____ mm Hg

4. _____ ; _____ mm Hg

5. _____ ; _____ mm Hg

6. _____ ; _____ mm Hg

7. _____ ; _____ mm Hg

Suspected abnormality:

Comments:

ANALYSIS

Rhythm: NSR

Pressure(s): RA

Waveform characteristics and measurements:

1.	*a* Wave	;	4	mm Hg
2.	*c* Wave	;		mm Hg
3.	*v* Wave	;	3	mm Hg
4.	Mean	;	2	mm Hg
5.		;		mm Hg
6.		;		mm Hg
7.		;		mm Hg

Suspected abnormality: Normal or hypovolemia

Comments: With an adequate cardiac output this low RA pressure would be considered normal, whereas with a low cardiac output this RA pressure would be considered abnormally low and indicate the need for increased volume.

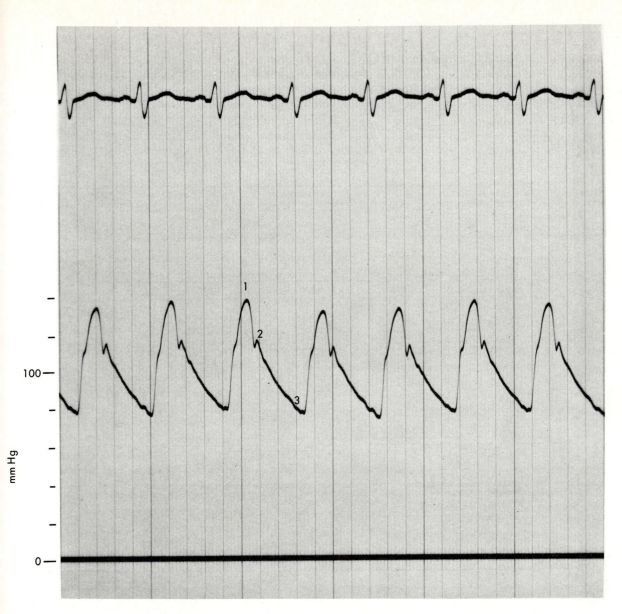

ANALYSIS

Rhythm:

Pressure(s):

Waveform characteristics and measurements:

1. _____ ; _____ mm Hg

2. _____ ; _____ mm Hg

3. _____ ; _____ mm Hg

4. _____ ; _____ mm Hg

5. _____ ; _____ mm Hg

6. _____ ; _____ mm Hg

7. _____ ; _____ mm Hg

Suspected abnormality:

Comments:

ANALYSIS

Rhythm: NSR

Pressure(s): Radial artery

Waveform characteristics and measurements:

1. _____Arterial systolic_____ ; _____135_____ mm Hg

2. _____Dicrotic notch_____ ; _____ mm Hg

3. _____Arterial end-diastolic_____ ; _____75_____ mm Hg

4. _____ ; _____ mm Hg

5. _____ ; _____ mm Hg

6. _____ ; _____ mm Hg

7. _____ ; _____ mm Hg

Suspected abnormality: Normal

Comments:

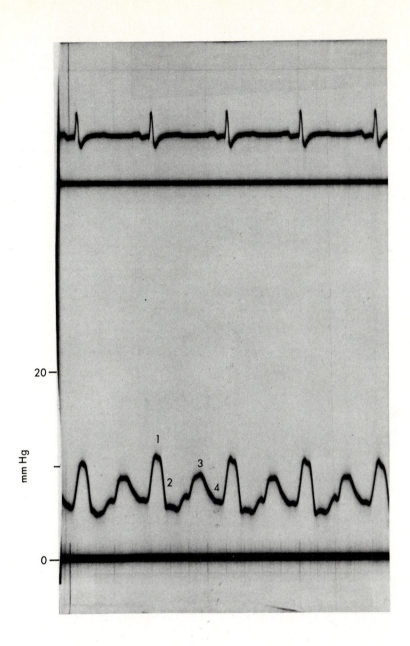

ANALYSIS

Rhythm:

Pressure(s):

Waveform characteristics and measurements:

1. _____ ; _____ mm Hg

2. _____ ; _____ mm Hg

3. _____ ; _____ mm Hg

4. _____ ; _____ mm Hg

5. _____ ; _____ mm Hg

6. _____ ; _____ mm Hg

7. _____ ; _____ mm Hg

Suspected abnormality:

Comments:

ANALYSIS

Rhythm: NSR

Pressure(s): PAW

Waveform characteristics and measurements:

1. _____ a Wave _____ ; _____ 10 _____ mm Hg

2. _____ x Descent _____ ; _____ mm Hg

3. _____ v Wave _____ ; _____ 8 _____ mm Hg

4. _____ y Descent _____ ; _____ mm Hg

5. _____ Mean _____ ; _____ 8 _____ mm Hg

6. _____ ; _____ mm Hg

7. _____ ; _____ mm Hg

Suspected abnormality: Normal

Comments:

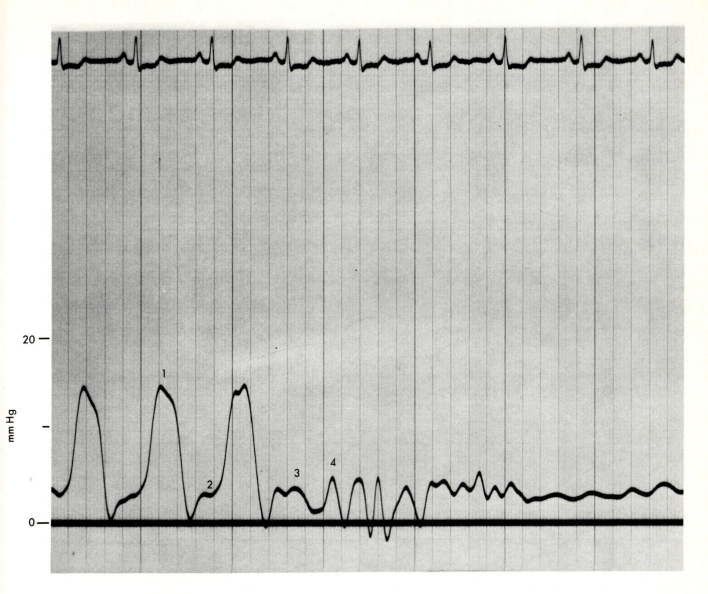

ANALYSIS

Rhythm:

Pressure(s):

Waveform characteristics and measurements:

1. _____ ; _____ mm Hg

2. _____ ; _____ mm Hg

3. _____ ; _____ mm Hg

4. _____ ; _____ mm Hg

5. _____ ; _____ mm Hg

6. _____ ; _____ mm Hg

7. _____ ; _____ mm Hg

Suspected abnormality:

Comments:

ANALYSIS

Rhythm: NSR

Pressure(s): RV to RA

Waveform characteristics and measurements:

1.	RV systolic	;	15	mm Hg
2.	RV end-diastolic	;	4	mm Hg
3.	RA *a* wave	;	4	mm Hg
4.	RA *v* wave	;	5	mm Hg
5.	RA mean	;	4	mm Hg
6.		;		mm Hg
7.		;		mm Hg

Suspected abnormality: Normal

Comments: The catheter is withdrawn from the RV into the RA. The RA pressure waveform becomes damped, most likely because of curling of the catheter in the RA with consequent pushing of the catheter tip against the atrial wall. When the catheter is resting in the PA, it forms a distinct curve. Frequently this curve is maintained, even when the catheter is withdrawn into another chamber.

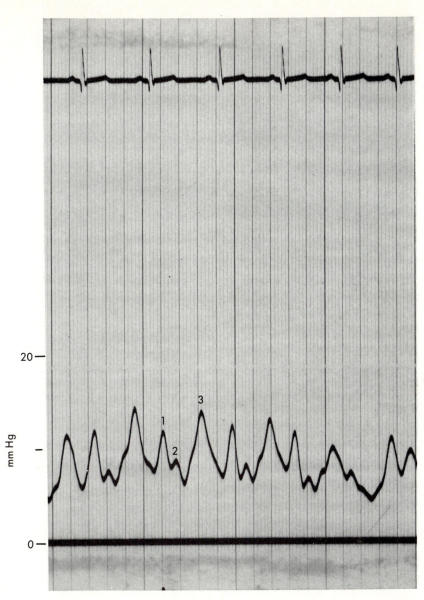

ANALYSIS

Rhythm:

Pressure(s):

Waveform characteristics and measurements:

1. _____ ; _____ mm Hg

2. _____ ; _____ mm Hg

3. _____ ; _____ mm Hg

4. _____ ; _____ mm Hg

5. _____ ; _____ mm Hg

6. _____ ; _____ mm Hg

7. _____ ; _____ mm Hg

Suspected abnormality:

Comments:

ANALYSIS

Rhythm: NSR

Pressure(s): PAW

Waveform characteristics and measurements:

1. _____ *a* Wave _____ ; _____ 12 _____ mm Hg
2. _____ *c* Wave _____ ; _____ mm Hg
3. _____ *v* Wave _____ ; _____ 12 _____ mm Hg
4. _____ Mean _____ ; _____ 9 _____ mm Hg
5. _____ ; _____ mm Hg
6. _____ ; _____ mm Hg
7. _____ ; _____ mm Hg

Suspected abnormality: Normal

Comments:

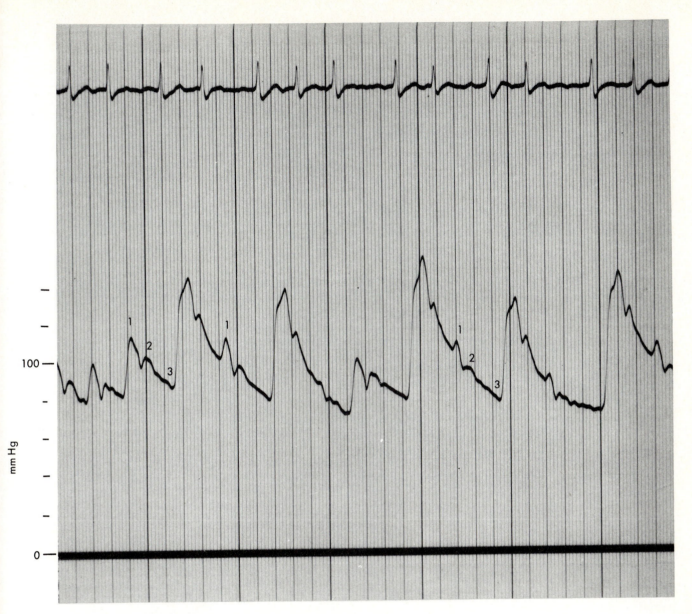

ANALYSIS

Rhythm:

Pressure(s):

Waveform characteristics and measurements:

1. _____ ; _____ mm Hg

2. _____ ; _____ mm Hg

3. _____ ; _____ mm Hg

4. _____ ; _____ mm Hg

5. _____ ; _____ mm Hg

6. _____ ; _____ mm Hg

7. _____ ; _____ mm Hg

Suspected abnormality:

Comments:

197

ANALYSIS

Rhythm: Atrial fibrillation

Pressure(s): Radial artery

Waveform characteristics and measurements:

1. _____Arterial systolic_____ ; _____100-145_____ mm Hg

2. _____Dicrotic notch_____ ; _____ mm Hg

3. _____Arterial end-diastolic_____ ; _____78_____ mm Hg

4. _____ ; _____ mm Hg

5. _____ ; _____ mm Hg

6. _____ ; _____ mm Hg

7. _____ ; _____ mm Hg

Suspected abnormality: Normal

Comments: Note the marked beat-to-beat pressure variation due to atrial fibrillation.

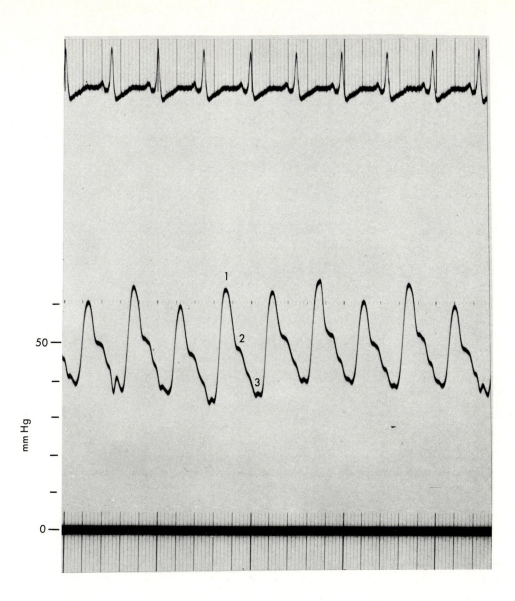

ANALYSIS

Rhythm:

Pressure(s):

Waveform characteristics and measurements:

1. _____ ; _____ mm Hg

2. _____ ; _____ mm Hg

3. _____ ; _____ mm Hg

4. _____ ; _____ mm Hg

5. _____ ; _____ mm Hg

6. _____ ; _____ mm Hg

7. _____ ; _____ mm Hg

Suspected abnormality:

Comments:

ANALYSIS

Rhythm: Sinus tachycardia

Pressure(s): PA

Waveform characteristics and measurements:

1.	PA systolic	;	62	mm Hg
2.	Dicrotic notch	;		mm Hg
3.	PA end-diastolic	;	38	mm Hg
4.		;		mm Hg
5.		;		mm Hg
6.		;		mm Hg
7.		;		mm Hg

Suspected abnormality: Pulmonary hypertension

Comments:

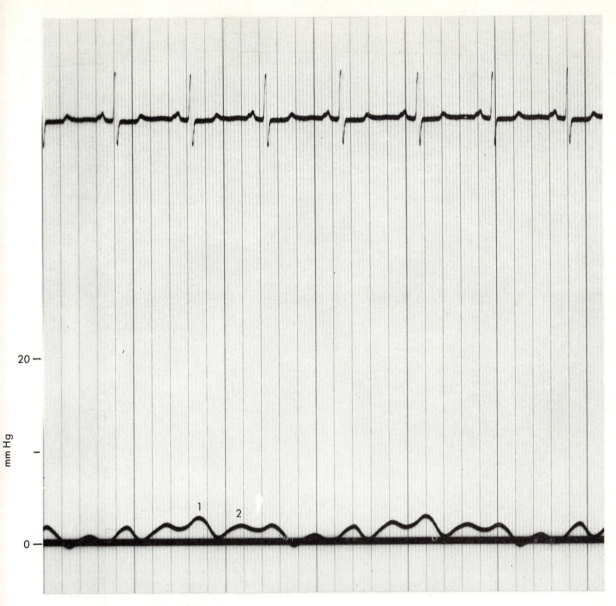

ANALYSIS

Rhythm:

Pressure(s):

Waveform characteristics and measurements:

1. _____ ; _____ mm Hg

2. _____ ; _____ mm Hg

3. _____ ; _____ mm Hg

4. _____ ; _____ mm Hg

5. _____ ; _____ mm Hg

6. _____ ; _____ mm Hg

7. _____ ; _____ mm Hg

Suspected abnormality:

Comments:

ANALYSIS

Rhythm: NSR

Pressure(s): RA

Waveform characteristics and measurements:

1. _____ *a* Wave _____ ; _____ 2 _____ mm Hg

2. _____ *v* Wave _____ ; _____ 1 _____ mm Hg

3. _____ Mean _____ ; _____ 1 _____ mm Hg

4. _____ ; _____ mm Hg

5. _____ ; _____ mm Hg

6. _____ ; _____ mm Hg

7. _____ ; _____ mm Hg

Suspected abnormality: Hypovolemia or incorrect transducer air-reference level

Comments:

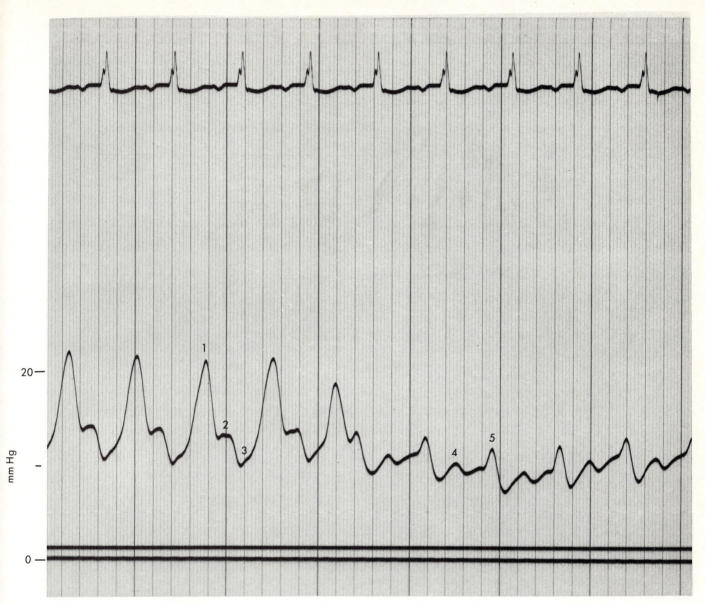

ANALYSIS

Rhythm:

Pressure(s):

Waveform characteristics and measurements:

1. _____ ; _____ mm Hg

2. _____ ; _____ mm Hg

3. _____ ; _____ mm Hg

4. _____ ; _____ mm Hg

5. _____ ; _____ mm Hg

6. _____ ; _____ mm Hg

7. _____ ; _____ mm Hg

Suspected abnormality:

Comments:

ANALYSIS

Rhythm: NSR

Pressure(s): PA to PAW

Waveform characteristics and measurements:

1.	PA systolic	;	22 mm Hg
2.	Dicrotic notch	;	mm Hg
3.	PA end-diastolic	;	10 mm Hg
4.	PAW *a* wave	;	10 mm Hg
5.	PAW *v* wave	;	12 mm Hg
6.	PAW mean	;	10 mm Hg
7.		;	mm Hg

Suspected abnormality: Normal

Comments: Note the similarity between the PAW pressure and the PAedp. Since the contour of the PAW pressure waveform is normal and correlates closely with the PAedp, it is prudent to monitor the PAedp as a reflection of the LVedp and thus minimize the number of balloon inflations.

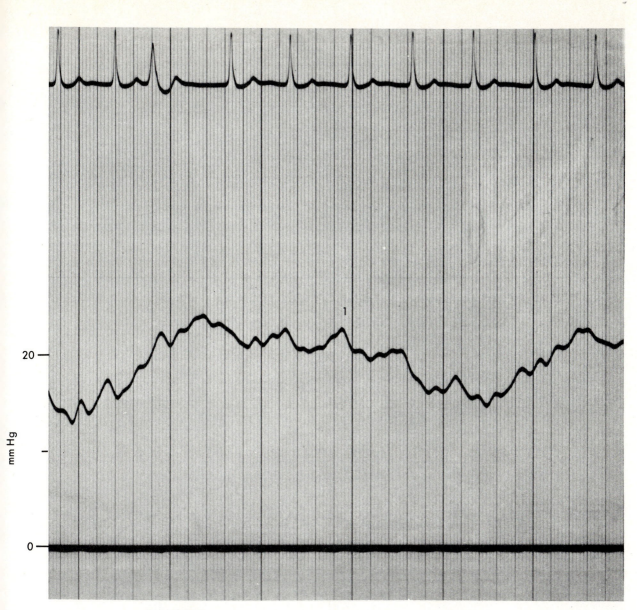

ANALYSIS

Rhythm:

Pressure(s):

Waveform characteristics and measurements:

1. _____ ; _____ mm Hg
2. _____ ; _____ mm Hg
3. _____ ; _____ mm Hg
4. _____ ; _____ mm Hg
5. _____ ; _____ mm Hg
6. _____ ; _____ mm Hg
7. _____ ; _____ mm Hg

Suspected abnormality:

Comments:

ANALYSIS

Rhythm: Atrial fibrillation with a PVC

Pressure(s): PAW

Waveform characteristics and measurements:

1. _____ v Wave _____ ; _____ 17 _____ mm Hg
2. _____ Mean _____ ; _____ 18 _____ mm Hg
3. _____ ; _____ mm Hg
4. _____ ; _____ mm Hg
5. _____ ; _____ mm Hg
6. _____ ; _____ mm Hg
7. _____ ; _____ mm Hg

Suspected abnormality: CHF

Comments: Note the lack of a waves due to atrial fibrillation. Normal respiratory variation is present.

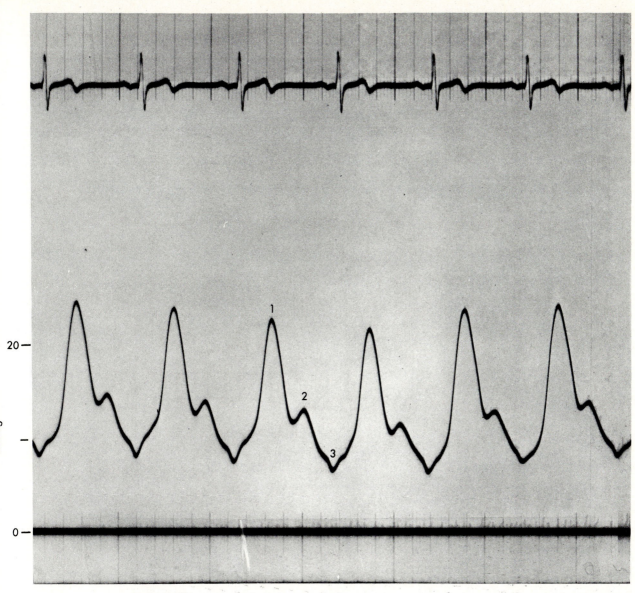

ANALYSIS

Rhythm:

Pressure(s):

Waveform characteristics and measurements:

1. _____ ; _____ mm Hg

2. _____ ; _____ mm Hg

3. _____ ; _____ mm Hg

4. _____ ; _____ mm Hg

5. _____ ; _____ mm Hg

6. _____ ; _____ mm Hg

7. _____ ; _____ mm Hg

Suspected abnormality:

Comments: 207

ANALYSIS

Rhythm: NSR

Pressure(s): PA

Waveform characteristics and measurements:

1.	PA systolic	;	24	mm Hg
2.	Dicrotic notch	;		mm Hg
3.	PA end-diastolic	;	9	mm Hg
4.		;		mm Hg
5.		;		mm Hg
6.		;		mm Hg
7.		;		mm Hg

Suspected abnormality: Normal

Comments:

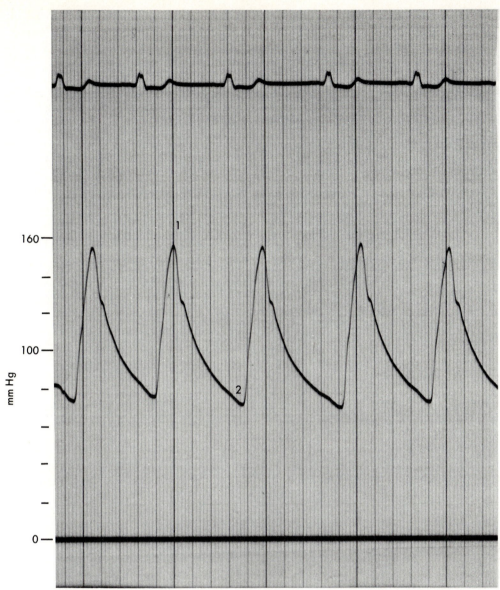

ANALYSIS

Rhythm:

Pressure(s):

Waveform characteristics and measurements:

1. _____ ; _____ mm Hg

2. _____ ; _____ mm Hg

3. _____ ; _____ mm Hg

4. _____ ; _____ mm Hg

5. _____ ; _____ mm Hg

6. _____ ; _____ mm Hg

7. _____ ; _____ mm Hg

Suspected abnormality:

Comments:

ANALYSIS

Rhythm: (?) Atrial fibrillation

Pressure(s): Radial artery

Waveform characteristics and measurements:

1. _____Arterial systolic_____ ; _____155_____ mm Hg
2. _____Arterial end-diastolic_____ ; _____70_____ mm Hg
3. _____ ; _____ mm Hg
4. _____ ; _____ mm Hg
5. _____ ; _____ mm Hg
6. _____ ; _____ mm Hg
7. _____ ; _____ mm Hg

Suspected abnormality: Mild aortic regurgitation

Comments: Note the rather wide pulse pressure (85 mm Hg) and poorly defined dicrotic notch seen in aortic regurgitation.

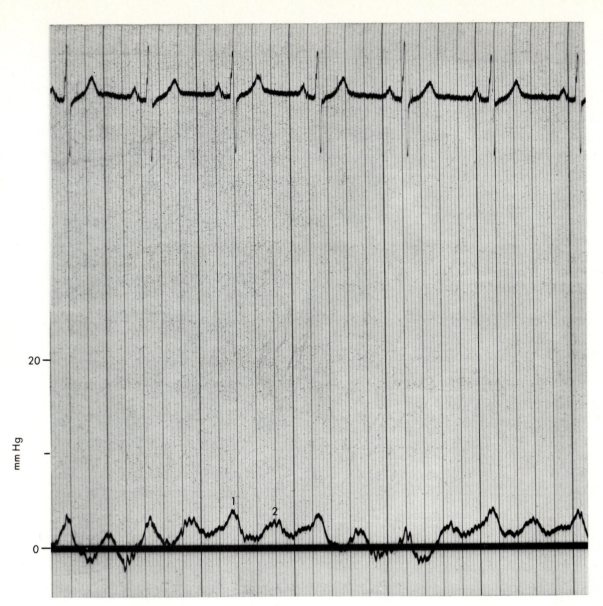

ANALYSIS

Rhythm:

Pressure(s):

Waveform characteristics and measurements:

1. _____ ; _____ mm Hg

2. _____ ; _____ mm Hg

3. _____ ; _____ mm Hg

4. _____ ; _____ mm Hg

5. _____ ; _____ mm Hg

6. _____ ; _____ mm Hg

7. _____ ; _____ mm Hg

Suspected abnormality:

Comments:

ANALYSIS

Rhythm: NSR

Pressure(s): RA

Waveform characteristics and measurements:

1. _____ *a* Wave _____ ; _____ 4 _____ mm Hg
2. _____ *v* Wave _____ ; _____ 2 _____ mm Hg
3. _____ ; _____ mm Hg
4. _____ ; _____ mm Hg
5. _____ ; _____ mm Hg
6. _____ ; _____ mm Hg
7. _____ ; _____ mm Hg

Suspected abnormality: Low normal

Comments:

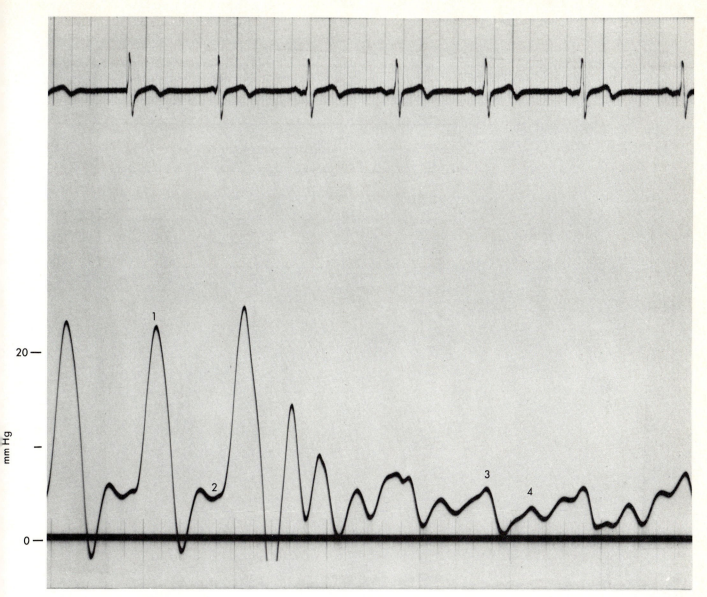

ANALYSIS

Rhythm:

Pressure(s):

Waveform characteristics and measurements:

1. _____ ; _____ mm Hg

2. _____ ; _____ mm Hg

3. _____ ; _____ mm Hg

4. _____ ; _____ mm Hg

5. _____ ; _____ mm Hg

6. _____ ; _____ mm Hg

7. _____ ; _____ mm Hg

Suspected abnormality:

Comments:

ANALYSIS

Rhythm: NSR

Pressure(s): RV to RA

Waveform characteristics and measurements:

1.	RV systolic	;	23	mm Hg
2.	RVedp	;	4	mm Hg
3.	RA *a* wave	;	6	mm Hg
4.	RA *v* wave	;	4	mm Hg
5.		;		mm Hg
6.		;		mm Hg
7.		;		mm Hg

Suspected abnormality: Normal

Comments:

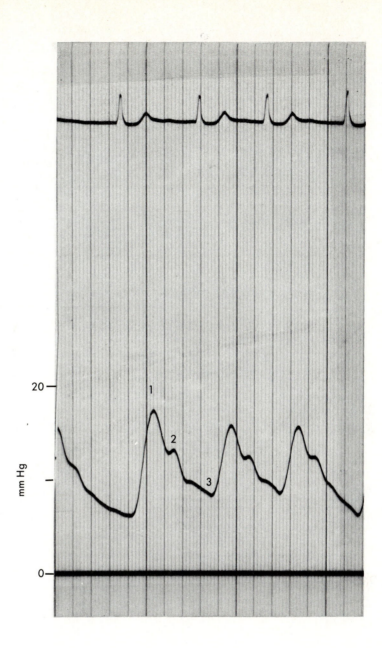

ANALYSIS

Rhythm:

Pressure(s):

Waveform characteristics and measurements:

    1. _____ ; _____ mm Hg

    2. _____ ; _____ mm Hg

    3. _____ ; _____ mm Hg

    4. _____ ; _____ mm Hg

    5. _____ ; _____ mm Hg

    6. _____ ; _____ mm Hg

    7. _____ ; _____ mm Hg

Suspected abnormality:

Comments:

ANALYSIS

Rhythm: Atrial fibrillation

Pressure(s): PA

Waveform characteristics and measurements:

1. _____ PA systolic _____ ; _____ 17 _____ mm Hg

2. _____ Dicrotic notch _____ ; _____ mm Hg

3. _____ PA end-diastolic _____ ; _____ 8 _____ mm Hg

4. _____ ; _____ mm Hg

5. _____ ; _____ mm Hg

6. _____ ; _____ mm Hg

7. _____ ; _____ mm Hg

Suspected abnormality: Normal

Comments:

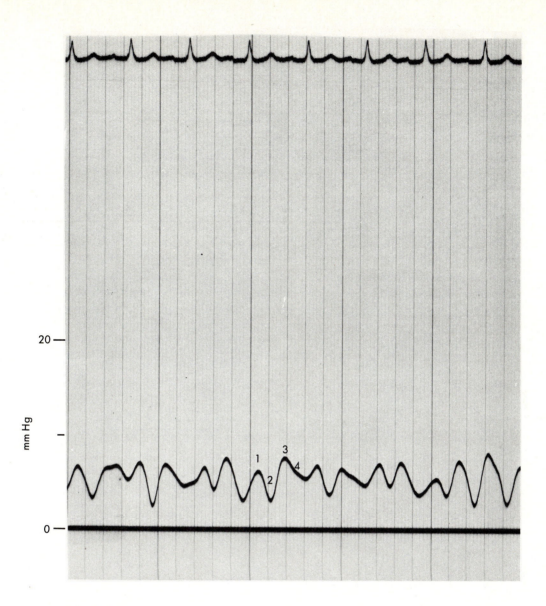

ANALYSIS

Rhythm:

Pressure(s):

Waveform characteristics and measurements:

1. _____ ; _____ mm Hg

2. _____ ; _____ mm Hg

3. _____ ; _____ mm Hg

4. _____ ; _____ mm Hg

5. _____ ; _____ mm Hg

6. _____ ; _____ mm Hg

7. _____ ; _____ mm Hg

Suspected abnormality:

Comments:

ANALYSIS

Rhythm: NSR

Pressure(s): PAW

Waveform characteristics and measurements:

1. _____ *a* Wave _____ ; _____ 7 _____ mm Hg
2. _____ *x* Descent _____ ; _____ mm Hg
3. _____ *v* Wave _____ ; _____ 7 _____ mm Hg
4. _____ *y* Descent _____ ; _____ mm Hg
5. _____ Mean _____ ; _____ 5 _____ mm Hg
6. _____ ; _____ mm Hg
7. _____ ; _____ mm Hg

Suspected abnormality: Normal

Comments:

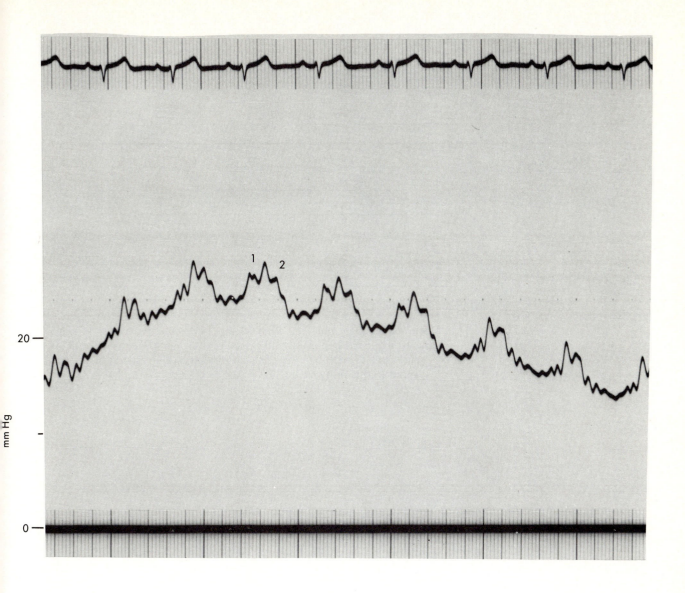

ANALYSIS

Rhythm:

Pressure(s):

Waveform characteristics and measurements:

1. _____ ; _____ mm Hg

2. _____ ; _____ mm Hg

3. _____ ; _____ mm Hg

4. _____ ; _____ mm Hg

5. _____ ; _____ mm Hg

6. _____ ; _____ mm Hg

7. _____ ; _____ mm Hg

Suspected abnormality:

Comments:

ANALYSIS

Rhythm: NSR

Pressure(s): PAW

Waveform characteristics and measurements:

1. _____ *a* Wave _____ ; _____ 23 _____ mm Hg

2. _____ *v* Wave _____ ; _____ 23 _____ mm Hg

3. _____ Mean _____ ; _____ 20 _____ mm Hg

4. _____ ; _____ mm Hg

5. _____ ; _____ mm Hg

6. _____ ; _____ mm Hg

7. _____ ; _____ mm Hg

Suspected abnormality: CHF

Comments: Since neither the *a* nor the *v* wave of this PAW pressure tracing is dominant or significantly elevated, it is accurate to use a mean of the PAW pressure rises to reflect LVedp. This also averages the respiratory changes that occur in this pressure tracing.

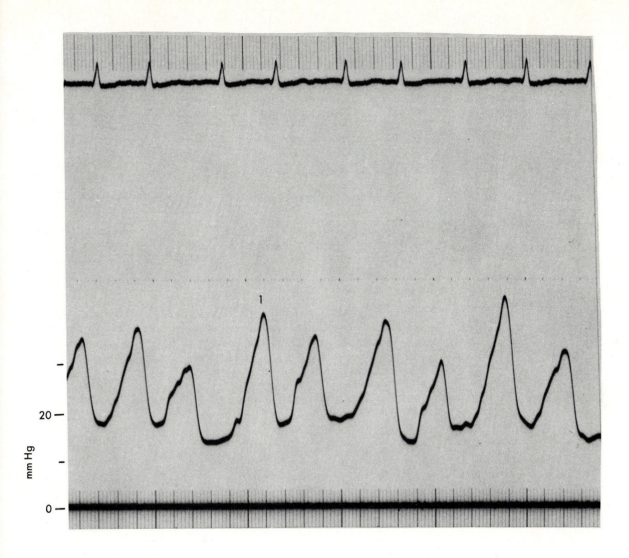

ANALYSIS

Rhythm:

Pressure(s):

Waveform characteristics and measurements:

1. _____ ; _____ mm Hg

2. _____ ; _____ mm Hg

3. _____ ; _____ mm Hg

4. _____ ; _____ mm Hg

5. _____ ; _____ mm Hg

6. _____ ; _____ mm Hg

7. _____ ; _____ mm Hg

Suspected abnormality:

Comments:

ANALYSIS

Rhythm: Atrial fibrillation

Pressure(s): PAW

Waveform characteristics and measurements:

1. _____ v Wave _____ ; _____ 37 _____ mm Hg

2. _____ ; _____ mm Hg

3. _____ ; _____ mm Hg

4. _____ ; _____ mm Hg

5. _____ ; _____ mm Hg

6. _____ ; _____ mm Hg

7. _____ ; _____ mm Hg

Suspected abnormality: Mitral regurgitation

Comments: With atrial fibrillation and loss of electrical atrial systole there is a corresponding loss of mechanical atrial systole; therefore there are no a waves in this PAW waveform. There is only a v wave for each QRS complex. In this case the v wave is moderately elevated with a rapid y descent due to mitral regurgitation.

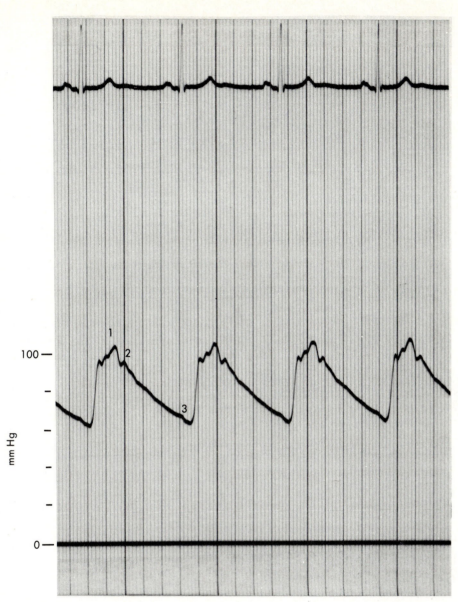

ANALYSIS

Rhythm:

Pressure(s):

Waveform characteristics and measurements:

1. _____ ; _____ mm Hg

2. _____ ; _____ mm Hg

3. _____ ; _____ mm Hg

4. _____ ; _____ mm Hg

5. _____ ; _____ mm Hg

6. _____ ; _____ mm Hg

7. _____ ; _____ mm Hg

Suspected abnormality:

Comments:

ANALYSIS

Rhythm: NSR

Pressure(s): Central arterial

Waveform characteristics and measurements:

1.	Arterial systolic	;	100	mm Hg
2.	Dicrotic notch	;		mm Hg
3.	Arterial end-diastolic	;	65	mm Hg
4.		;		mm Hg
5.		;		mm Hg
6.		;		mm Hg
7.		;		mm Hg

Suspected abnormality: Hypotension

Comments:

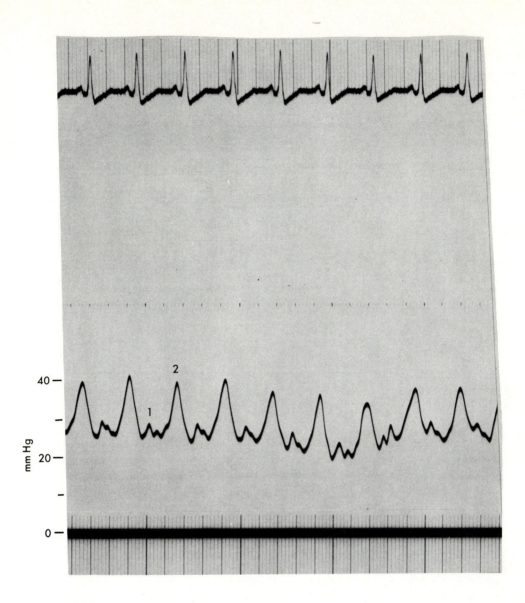

ANALYSIS

Rhythm:

Pressure(s):

Waveform characteristics and measurements:

1. _____ ; _____ mm Hg

2. _____ ; _____ mm Hg

3. _____ ; _____ mm Hg

4. _____ ; _____ mm Hg

5. _____ ; _____ mm Hg

6. _____ ; _____ mm Hg

7. _____ ; _____ mm Hg

Suspected abnormality:

Comments:

ANALYSIS   –

Rhythm: Sinus tachycardia

Pressure(s): PAW

Waveform characteristics and measurements:

1. _____ *a* Wave _____ ; _____ 27 _____ mm Hg
2. _____ *v* Wave _____ ; _____ 38 _____ mm Hg
3. _____ ; _____ mm Hg
4. _____ ; _____ mm Hg
5. _____ ; _____ mm Hg
6. _____ ; _____ mm Hg
7. _____ ; _____ mm Hg

Suspected abnormality: Mitral regurgitation with LV failure

Comments: The dominant and elevated *v* wave of 38 mm Hg suggests moderate mitral regurgitation. The *a* wave of 25 mm Hg indicates LV failure. In this case the mitral regurgitation may be functional secondary to LV failure with dilatation.

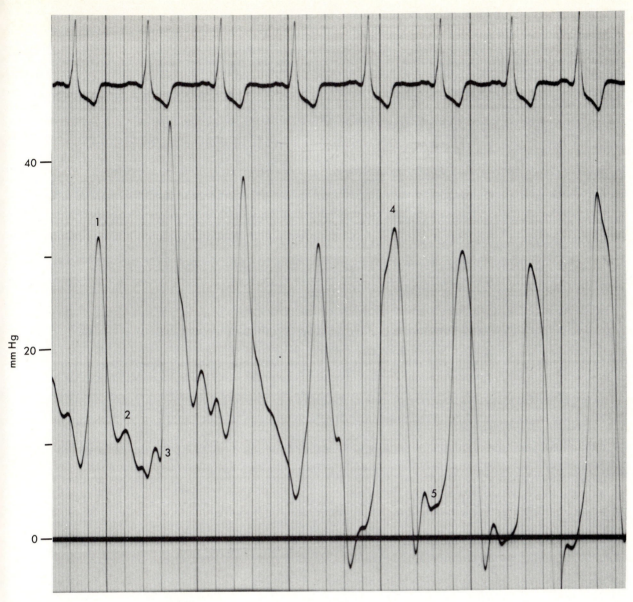

ANALYSIS

Rhythm:

Pressure(s):

Waveform characteristics and measurements:

1. _____ ; _____ mm Hg

2. _____ ; _____ mm Hg

3. _____ ; _____ mm Hg

4. _____ ; _____ mm Hg

5. _____ ; _____ mm Hg

6. _____ ; _____ mm Hg

7. _____ ; _____ mm Hg

Suspected abnormality:

Comments:

ANALYSIS

Rhythm: NSR

Pressure(s): PA to RV

Waveform characteristics and measurements:

1.	PA systolic	;	35	mm Hg
2.	Dicrotic notch	;		mm Hg
3.	PA end-diastolic	;	10	mm Hg
4.	RV systolic	;	34	mm Hg
5.	RV end-diastolic	;	2	mm Hg
6.		;		mm Hg
7.		;		mm Hg

Suspected abnormality: Mild pulmonary hypertension

Comments: Note the similarity between the PA and RV systolic pressures and the discrepancy between the PA and RV diastolic pressures. If only the systolic digital value were being monitored in this patient, it would be possible to overlook the fact that the catheter tip has withdrawn back into the RV, a potentially hazardous situation. Monitoring the contour of the pressure waveform on the oscilloscope is essential to accurately identify the location of the pressure. Additionally, the digital mode selection should be set at *diastole* rather than *systole*, since it is that value which reflects the LVedp, and it is that value which will change immediately if the catheter tip falls into the RV.

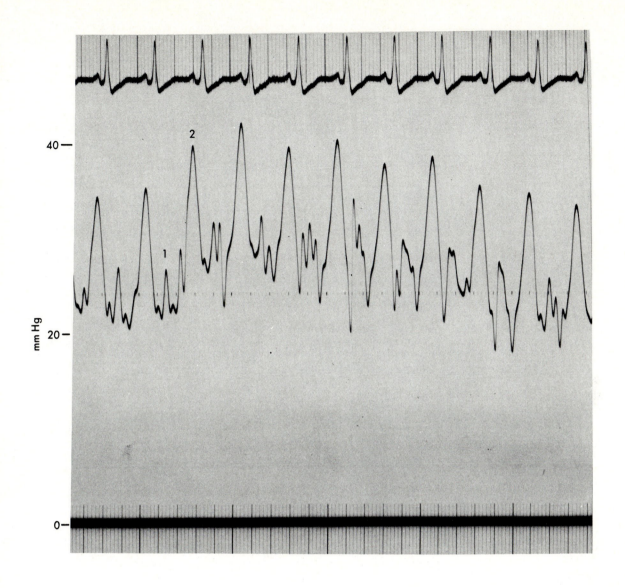

ANALYSIS

Rhythm:

Pressure(s):

Waveform characteristics and measurements:

1. _____ ; _____ mm Hg

2. _____ ; _____ mm Hg

3. _____ ; _____ mm Hg

4. _____ ; _____ mm Hg

5. _____ ; _____ mm Hg

6. _____ ; _____ mm Hg

7. _____ ; _____ mm Hg

Suspected abnormality:

Comments:

ANALYSIS

Rhythm: Sinus tachycardia

Pressure(s): PAW

Waveform characteristics and measurements:

1. _____ *a* Wave _____ ; _____ 30 _____ mm Hg
2. _____ *v* Wave _____ ; _____ 38 _____ mm Hg
3. _____ ; _____ mm Hg
4. _____ ; _____ mm Hg
5. _____ ; _____ mm Hg
6. _____ ; _____ mm Hg
7. _____ ; _____ mm Hg

Suspected abnormality: LV Failure with mitral regurgitation

Comments: LV failure with compensatory dilatation of the ventricle commonly produces some mitral regurgitation, as evidenced in this patient with a dominant, elevated *v* wave of 38 mm Hg. The elevated *a* wave of 30 mm Hg suggests severe LV failure.

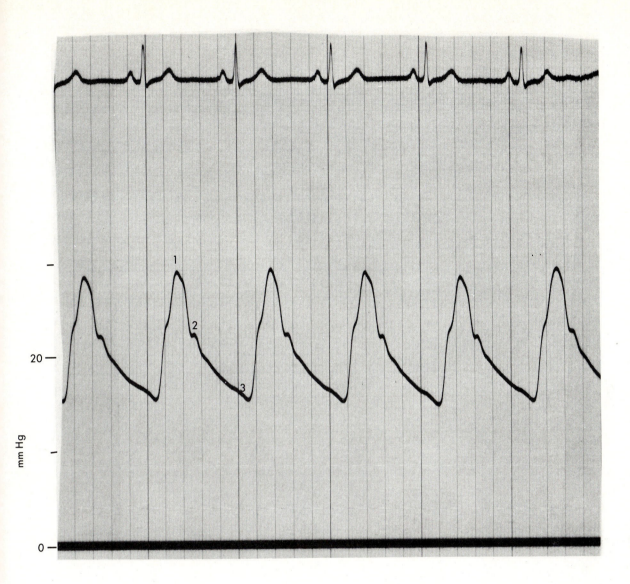

ANALYSIS

Rhythm:

Pressure(s):

Waveform characteristics and measurements:

1. _____ ; _____ mm Hg

2. _____ ; _____ mm Hg

3. _____ ; _____ mm Hg

4. _____ ; _____ mm Hg

5. _____ ; _____ mm Hg

6. _____ ; _____ mm Hg

7. _____ ; _____ mm Hg

Suspected abnormality:

Comments:

ANALYSIS

Rhythm: NSR

Pressure(s): PA

Waveform characteristics and measurements:

1. _____ PA systolic _____ ; _____ 28 _____ mm Hg
2. _____ Dicrotic notch _____ ; _____ mm Hg
3. _____ PA end-diastolic _____ ; _____ 15 _____ mm Hg
4. _____ ; _____ mm Hg
5. _____ ; _____ mm Hg
6. _____ ; _____ mm Hg
7. _____ ; _____ mm Hg

Suspected abnormality: Mild CHF

Comments:

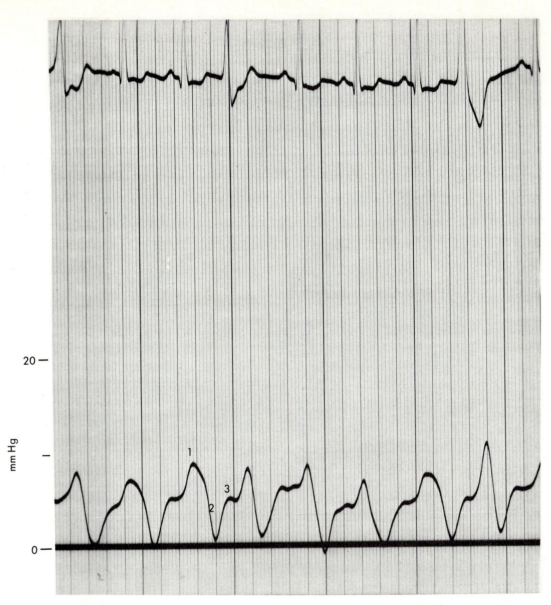

ANALYSIS

Rhythm:

Pressure(s):

Waveform characteristics and measurements:

1. _____ ; _____ mm Hg

2. _____ ; _____ mm Hg

3. _____ ; _____ mm Hg

4. _____ ; _____ mm Hg

5. _____ ; _____ mm Hg

6. _____ ; _____ mm Hg

7. _____ ; _____ mm Hg

Suspected abnormality:

Comments:

ANALYSIS

Rhythm: NSR with PVCs

Pressure(s): RA

Waveform characteristics and measurements:

1. _____ *a* Wave _____ ; ___ 9 ___ mm Hg
2. _____ *x* Descent _____ ; _____ mm Hg
3. _____ *v* Wave _____ ; ___ 6 ___ mm Hg
4. _____ Mean _____ ; ___ 5 ___ mm Hg
5. _____ ; _____ mm Hg
6. _____ ; _____ mm Hg
7. _____ ; _____ mm Hg

Suspected abnormality: Normal

Comments:

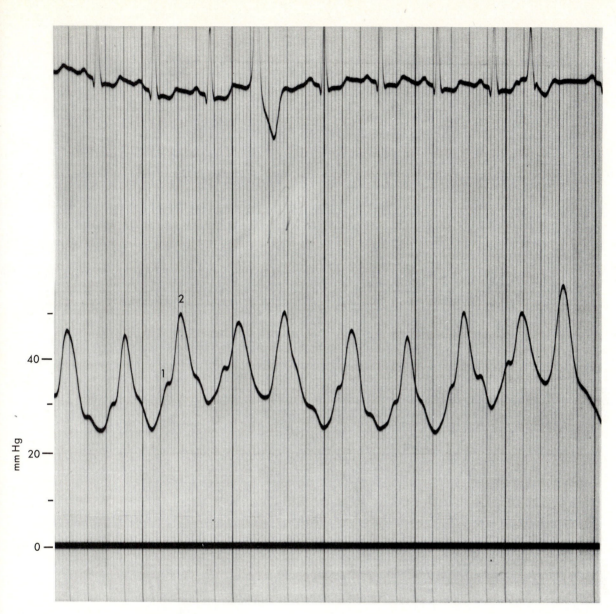

ANALYSIS

Rhythm:

Pressure(s):

Waveform characteristics and measurements:

1. _____ ; _____ mm Hg

2. _____ ; _____ mm Hg

3. _____ ; _____ mm Hg

4. _____ ; _____ mm Hg

5. _____ ; _____ mm Hg

6. _____ ; _____ mm Hg

7. _____ ; _____ mm Hg

Suspected abnormality:

Comments:

ANALYSIS

Rhythm: Sinus tachycardia with PVC and APC

Pressure(s): PAW

Waveform characteristics and measurements:

1. _____ *a* Wave _____ ; _____ 35 _____ mm Hg

2. _____ *v* Wave _____ ; _____ 48 _____ mm Hg

3. _____ ; _____ mm Hg

4. _____ ; _____ mm Hg

5. _____ ; _____ mm Hg

6. _____ ; _____ mm Hg

7. _____ ; _____ mm Hg

Suspected abnormality: Mitral regurgitation with LV failure

Comments: The dominant and elevated *v* wave of 48 mm Hg is due to mitral regurgitation; the *a* wave of 35 mm Hg suggests severe LV failure.

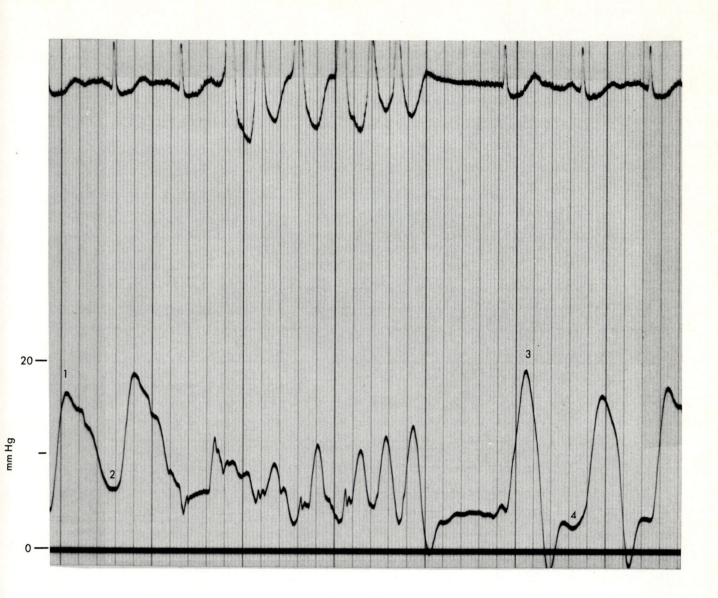

ANALYSIS

Rhythm:

Pressure(s):

Waveform characteristics and measurements:

1. _____ ; _____ mm Hg

2. _____ ; _____ mm Hg

3. _____ ; _____ mm Hg

4. _____ ; _____ mm Hg

5. _____ ; _____ mm Hg

6. _____ ; _____ mm Hg

7. _____ ; _____ mm Hg

Suspected abnormality:

Comments:

ANALYSIS

Rhythm: NSR with six-beat run of VT

Pressure(s): PA to RV

Waveform characteristics and measurements:

1.	PA systolic	;	19	mm Hg
2.	PA end-diastolic	;	7	mm Hg
3.	RV systolic	;	19	mm Hg
4.	RV end-diastolic	;	3	mm Hg
5.		;		mm Hg
6.		;		mm Hg
7.		;		mm Hg

Suspected abnormality: Normal

Comments: The catheter tip has fallen from the PA into the RV, causing a brief run of VT. Repositioning of the catheter is necessary to prevent the occurrence of further ventricular arrhythmias. Note the similarity between the PA and RV systolic pressures but the disparity in the diastolic values with the RV diastolic pressure falling below baseline.

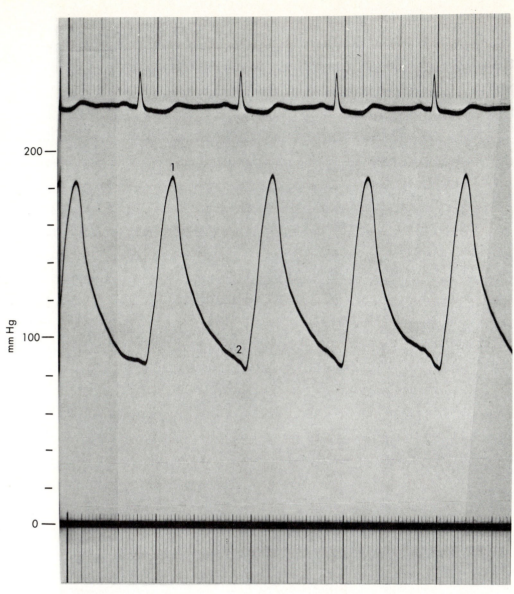

ANALYSIS

Rhythm:

Pressure(s):

Waveform characteristics and measurements:

1. _____ ; _____ mm Hg

2. _____ ; _____ mm Hg

3. _____ ; _____ mm Hg

4. _____ ; _____ mm Hg

5. _____ ; _____ mm Hg

6. _____ ; _____ mm Hg

7. _____ ; _____ mm Hg

Suspected abnormality:

Comments:

ANALYSIS

Rhythm: NSR

Pressure(s): Radial artery

Waveform characteristics and measurements:

1. _____Arterial systolic_____ ; _____180_____ mm Hg

2. _____Arterial end-diastolic_____ ; _____85_____ mm Hg

3. _____ ; _____ mm Hg

4. _____ ; _____ mm Hg

5. _____ ; _____ mm Hg

6. _____ ; _____ mm Hg

7. _____ ; _____ mm Hg

Suspected abnormality: Aortic regurgitation

Comments: Note the wide pulse pressure and absent dicrotic notch, which are indicative of aortic regurgitation.

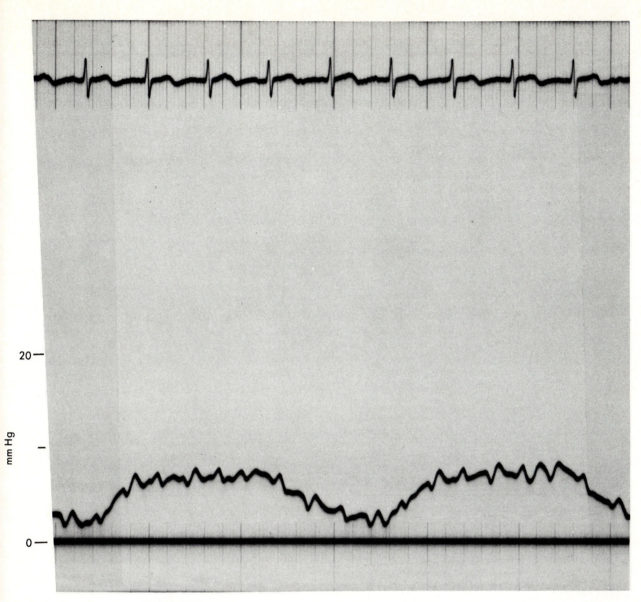

ANALYSIS

Rhythm:

Pressure(s):

Waveform characteristics and measurements:

1. _____ ; _____ mm Hg
2. _____ ; _____ mm Hg
3. _____ ; _____ mm Hg
4. _____ ; _____ mm Hg
5. _____ ; _____ mm Hg
6. _____ ; _____ mm Hg
7. _____ ; _____ mm Hg

Suspected abnormality:

Comments:

ANALYSIS

Rhythm: Regular supraventricular tachycardia

Pressure(s): PAW

Waveform characteristics and measurements:

1. _____Mean_____ ; _____6_____ mm Hg

2. _____ ; _____ mm Hg

3. _____ ; _____ mm Hg

4. _____ ; _____ mm Hg

5. _____ ; _____ mm Hg

6. _____ ; _____ mm Hg

7. _____ ; _____ mm Hg

Suspected abnormality: Normal

Comments: Note the normal respiratory variation.

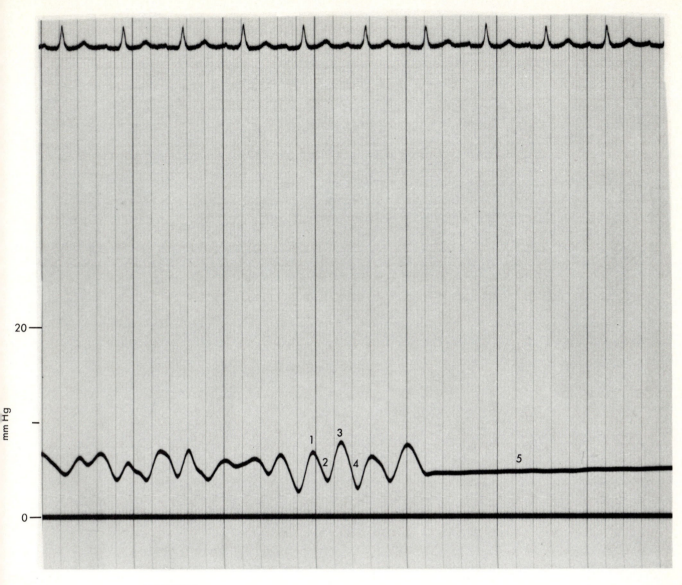

ANALYSIS

Rhythm:

Pressure(s):

Waveform characteristics and measurements:

1. _____ ; _____ mm Hg

2. _____ ; _____ mm Hg

3. _____ ; _____ mm Hg

4. _____ ; _____ mm Hg

5. _____ ; _____ mm Hg

6. _____ ; _____ mm Hg

7. _____ ; _____ mm Hg

Suspected abnormality:

Comments:

ANALYSIS

Rhythm: NSR

Pressure(s): RA

Waveform characteristics and measurements:

1.	_a_ Wave	;	6	mm Hg
2.	_x_ Descent	;		mm Hg
3.	v Wave	;	6	mm Hg
4.	_y_ Descent	;		mm Hg
5.	Electrical mean	;	5	mm Hg
6.		;		mm Hg
7.		;		mm Hg

Suspected abnormality: Normal

Comments:

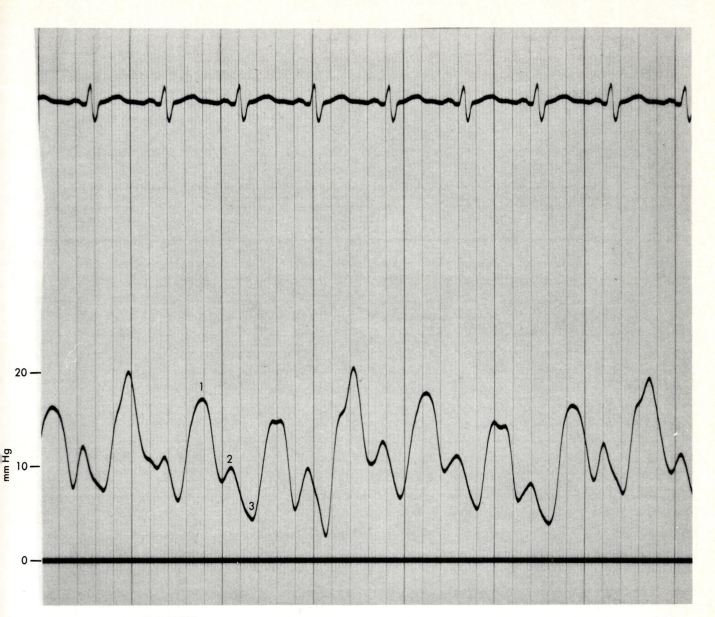

ANALYSIS

Rhythm:

Pressure(s):

Waveform characteristics and measurements:

1. _____ ; _____ mm Hg

2. _____ ; _____ mm Hg

3. _____ ; _____ mm Hg

4. _____ ; _____ mm Hg

5. _____ ; _____ mm Hg

6. _____ ; _____ mm Hg

7. _____ ; _____ mm Hg

Suspected abnormality:

Comments:

ANALYSIS

Rhythm: NSR

Pressure(s): PA

Waveform characteristics and measurements:

1. _____ PA systolic _____ ; _____ 18 _____ mm Hg

2. _____ Dicrotic notch _____ ; _____ mm Hg

3. _____ PA end-diastolic _____ ; _____ 6 _____ mm Hg

4. _____ ; _____ mm Hg

5. _____ ; _____ mm Hg

6. _____ ; _____ mm Hg

7. _____ ; _____ mm Hg

Suspected abnormality: Normal

Comments: Note the variation in pressure value and contour during normal respiration.

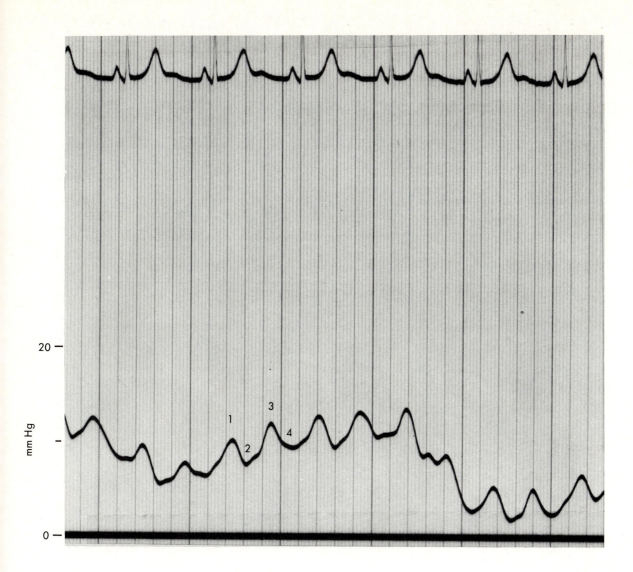

ANALYSIS

Rhythm:

Pressure(s):

Waveform characteristics and measurements:

1. _____ ; _____ mm Hg

2. _____ ; _____ mm Hg

3. _____ ; _____ mm Hg

4. _____ ; _____ mm Hg

5. _____ ; _____ mm Hg

6. _____ ; _____ mm Hg

7. _____ ; _____ mm Hg

Suspected abnormality:

Comments:

ANALYSIS

Rhythm: NSR

Pressure(s): PAW

Waveform characteristics and measurements:

1. _____ a Wave _____ ; _____ 10 _____ mm Hg
2. _____ x Descent _____ ; _____ mm Hg
3. _____ v Wave _____ ; _____ 10 _____ mm Hg
4. _____ y Descent _____ ; _____ mm Hg
5. _____ Mean _____ ; _____ 8 _____ mm Hg
6. _____ ; _____ mm Hg
7. _____ ; _____ mm Hg

Suspected abnormality: Normal

Comments:

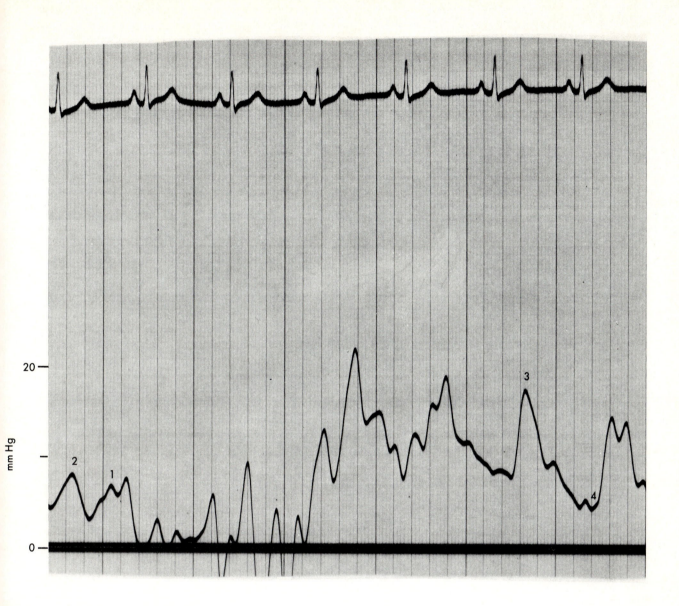

ANALYSIS

Rhythm:

Pressure(s):

Waveform characteristics and measurements:

1. _____ ; _____ mm Hg

2. _____ ; _____ mm Hg

3. _____ ; _____ mm Hg

4. _____ ; _____ mm Hg

5. _____ ; _____ mm Hg

6. _____ ; _____ mm Hg

7. _____ ; _____ mm Hg

Suspected abnormality:

Comments:

ANALYSIS

Rhythm: NSR

Pressure(s): PAW to PA

Waveform characteristics and measurements:

1. _____ PAW v wave _____ ; _____ 7 _____ mm Hg

2. _____ PAW a wave _____ ; _____ 7 _____ mm Hg

3. _____ PA systolic _____ ; _____ 19 _____ mm Hg

4. _____ PA end-diastolic _____ ; _____ 7 _____ mm Hg

5. _____ ; _____ mm Hg

6. _____ ; _____ mm Hg

7. _____ ; _____ mm Hg

Suspected abnormality: Normal

Comments: Note the correlation between the PAW and PAedp. The very low pressure oscillations between the PAW and PA waveforms are probably caused by handling of the catheter.

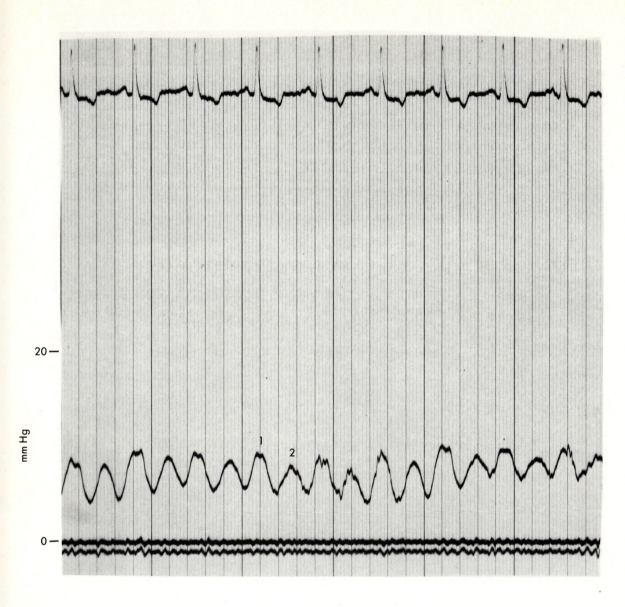

ANALYSIS

Rhythm:

Pressure(s):

Waveform characteristics and measurements:

1. _____ ; _____ mm Hg

2. _____ ; _____ mm Hg

3. _____ ; _____ mm Hg

4. _____ ; _____ mm Hg

5. _____ ; _____ mm Hg

6. _____ ; _____ mm Hg

7. _____ ; _____ mm Hg

Suspected abnormality:

Comments:

ANALYSIS

Rhythm: NSR

Pressure(s): RA

Waveform characteristics and measurements:

1.	_a_ Wave	;	8	mm Hg
2.	_v_ Wave	;	7	mm Hg
3.	Mean	;	6	mm Hg
4.		;		mm Hg
5.		;		mm Hg
6.		;		mm Hg
7.		;		mm Hg

Suspected abnormality: Normal

Comments: Note the lack of respiratory variation in this RA pressure due to momentary suspension of respirations at the end of expiration.

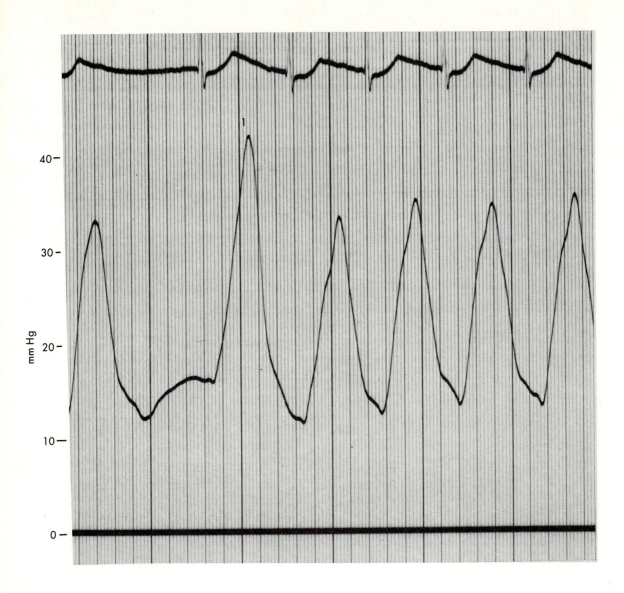

ANALYSIS

Rhythm:

Pressure(s):

Waveform characteristics and measurements:

1. _____ ; _____ mm Hg

2. _____ ; _____ mm Hg

3. _____ ; _____ mm Hg

4. _____ ; _____ mm Hg

5. _____ ; _____ mm Hg

6. _____ ; _____ mm Hg

7. _____ ; _____ mm Hg

Suspected abnormality:

Comments:

ANALYSIS

Rhythm: Nodal

Pressure(s): PAW

Waveform characteristics and measurements:

1. _____ *v* Wave _____ ; _____ 35 _____ mm Hg

2. _____ ; _____ mm Hg

3. _____ ; _____ mm Hg

4. _____ ; _____ mm Hg

5. _____ ; _____ mm Hg

6. _____ ; _____ mm Hg

7. _____ ; _____ mm Hg

Suspected abnormality: Severe mitral regurgitation

Comments: Note the increase in the size of the *v* wave, reflecting an increased regurgitant volume following a prolonged RR interval.

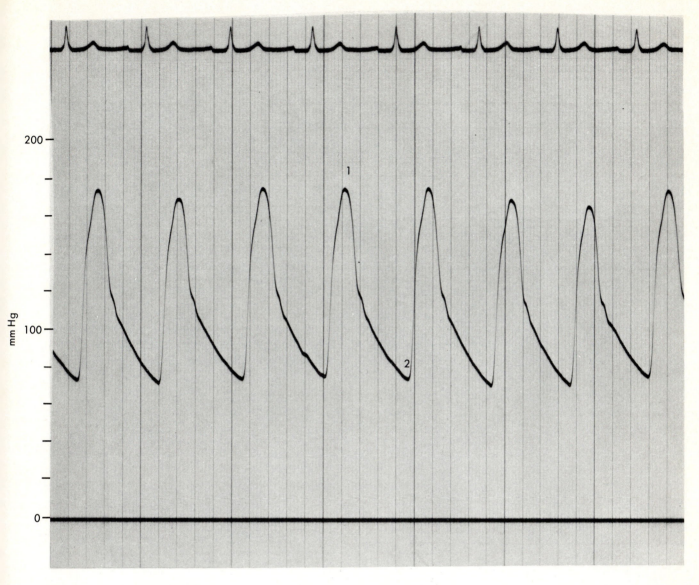

ANALYSIS

Rhythm:

Pressure(s):

Waveform characteristics and measurements:

1. _____ ; _____ mm Hg

2. _____ ; _____ mm Hg

3. _____ ; _____ mm Hg

4. _____ ; _____ mm Hg

5. _____ ; _____ mm Hg

6. _____ ; _____ mm Hg

7. _____ ; _____ mm Hg

Suspected abnormality:

Comments:

ANALYSIS

Rhythm: NSR

Pressure(s): Radial artery

Waveform characteristics and measurements:

1.	Arterial systolic	;	178	mm Hg
2.	Arterial end-diastolic	;	72	mm Hg
3.		;		mm Hg
4.		;		mm Hg
5.		;		mm Hg
6.		;		mm Hg
7.		;		mm Hg

Suspected abnormality: Aortic regurgitation

Comments: The wide pulse pressure (106 mm Hg) reflects a large stroke volume. This is due to the increased LV diastolic volume (the regurgitant volume plus the volume filled from the LA). The lack of a sharp dicrotic notch is due to the lack of complete closure of the aortic valve.

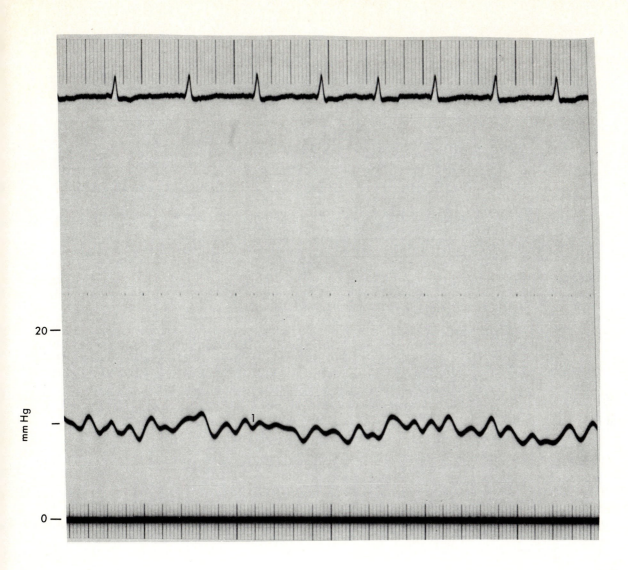

ANALYSIS

Rhythm:

Pressure(s):

Waveform characteristics and measurements:

1. _____ ; _____ mm Hg

2. _____ ; _____ mm Hg

3. _____ ; _____ mm Hg

4. _____ ; _____ mm Hg

5. _____ ; _____ mm Hg

6. _____ ; _____ mm Hg

7. _____ ; _____ mm Hg

Suspected abnormality:

Comments:

ANALYSIS

Rhythm: Atrial fibrillation

Pressure(s): RA

Waveform characteristics and measurements:

1. _____Fibrillatory waves_____ ; _____ mm Hg
2. _____Mean_____ ; _____10_____ mm Hg
3. _____ ; _____ mm Hg
4. _____ ; _____ mm Hg
5. _____ ; _____ mm Hg
6. _____ ; _____ mm Hg
7. _____ ; _____ mm Hg

Suspected abnormality: Normal or mild RV failure

Comments: With atrial fibrillation and a lack of atrial systole, we can expect to see only a v wave for each QRS complex. The numerous small pressure waves reflect fibrillatory activity of the atrium. Identification of the v wave is difficult but is hemodynamically insignificant, since all pressure fluctuations are essentially equal, resulting in a mean RA pressure of approximately 10 mm Hg—somewhat elevated.

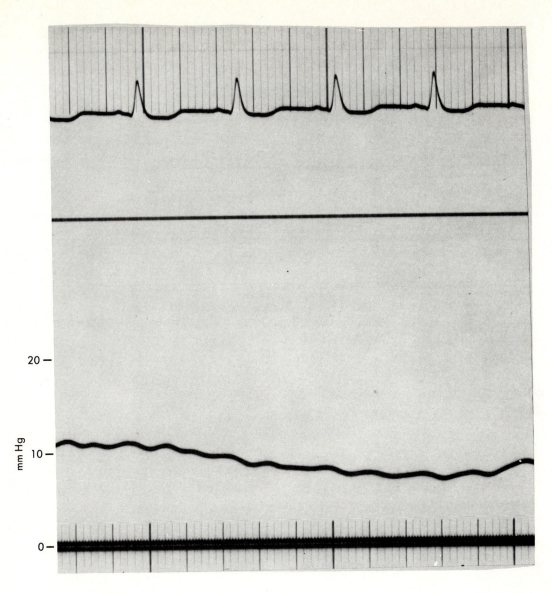

ANALYSIS

Rhythm:

Pressure(s):

Waveform characteristics and measurements:

1. _____ ; _____ mm Hg
2. _____ ; _____ mm Hg
3. _____ ; _____ mm Hg
4. _____ ; _____ mm Hg
5. _____ ; _____ mm Hg
6. _____ ; _____ mm Hg
7. _____ ; _____ mm Hg

Suspected abnormality:

Comments:

ANALYSIS

Rhythm: NSR

Pressure(s): (?)

Waveform characteristics and measurements:

1. _____ ; _____ mm Hg

2. _____ ; _____ mm Hg

3. _____ ; _____ mm Hg

4. _____ ; _____ mm Hg

5. _____ ; _____ mm Hg

6. _____ ; _____ mm Hg

7. _____ ; _____ mm Hg

Suspected abnormality:

Comments: This very damped pressure is unidentifiable and inaccurate. After deflation of the balloon to ensure that it is not wedged, the catheter should be aspirated and flushed.

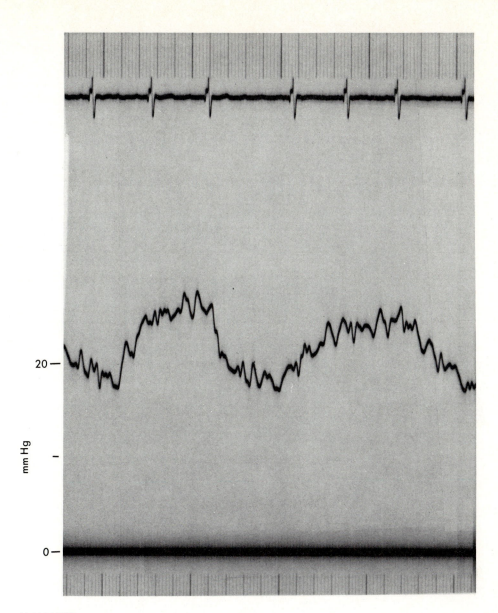

ANALYSIS

Rhythm:

Pressure(s):

Waveform characteristics and measurements:

1. _____ ; _____ mm Hg

2. _____ ; _____ mm Hg

3. _____ ; _____ mm Hg

4. _____ ; _____ mm Hg

5. _____ ; _____ mm Hg

6. _____ ; _____ mm Hg

7. _____ ; _____ mm Hg

Suspected abnormality:

Comments:

ANALYSIS

Rhythm: Atrial fibrillation

Pressure(s): PAW

Waveform characteristics and measurements:

1. _____Mean_____ ; _____22_____ mm Hg
2. _____ ; _____ mm Hg
3. _____ ; _____ mm Hg
4. _____ ; _____ mm Hg
5. _____ ; _____ mm Hg
6. _____ ; _____ mm Hg
7. _____ ; _____ mm Hg

Suspected abnormality: CHF

Comments: Because of atrial fibrillation, there are no *a* waves in this PAW pressure
waveform. The presence of numerous fibrillatory waves makes it difficult
to identify the *v* wave. If, by repositioning, it is impossible to obtain a better
PAW waveform, the mean of this pressure tracing can be used to reflect
the LVedp. In this case the PAW mean pressure is elevated (22 mm Hg),
indicating LV failure.

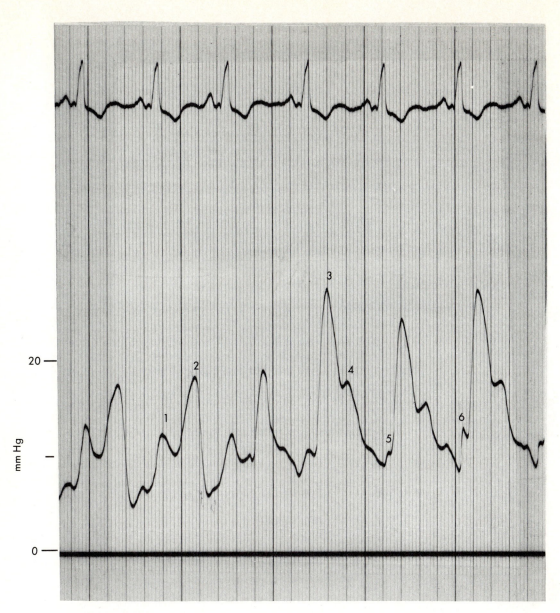

ANALYSIS

Rhythm:

Pressure(s):

Waveform characteristics and measurements:

1. _____ ; _____ mm Hg
2. _____ ; _____ mm Hg
3. _____ ; _____ mm Hg
4. _____ ; _____ mm Hg
5. _____ ; _____ mm Hg
6. _____ ; _____ mm Hg
7. _____ ; _____ mm Hg

Suspected abnormality:

Comments:

ANALYSIS

Rhythm: NSR

Pressure(s): PAW to PA

Waveform characteristics and measurements:

1.	PAW *a* wave	;	13	mm Hg
2.	PAW *v* wave	;	20	mm Hg
3.	PA systolic	;	27	mm Hg
4.	Dicrotic notch	;		mm Hg
5.	PA end-diastolic	;	12	mm Hg
6.	*a* Wave	;	11	mm Hg
7.		;		mm Hg

Suspected abnormality: Mild mitral regurgitation

Comments: The dominant and elevated PAW *v* wave of 20 mm Hg indicates mild regurgitation of blood through the somewhat incompetent mitral valve during systole. The rapid *y* descent is another indication of mitral regurgitation and is due to the enhanced emptying of the LA through the mitral valve. The slight elevation of the PAW *a* wave (13 mm Hg) indicates very mild LV failure. Waveform characteristic no. 6 may be the *a* wave of the PAW reflected back in the PA pressure waveform. Note its correlation to the P wave of the ECG and the PAW *a* wave.

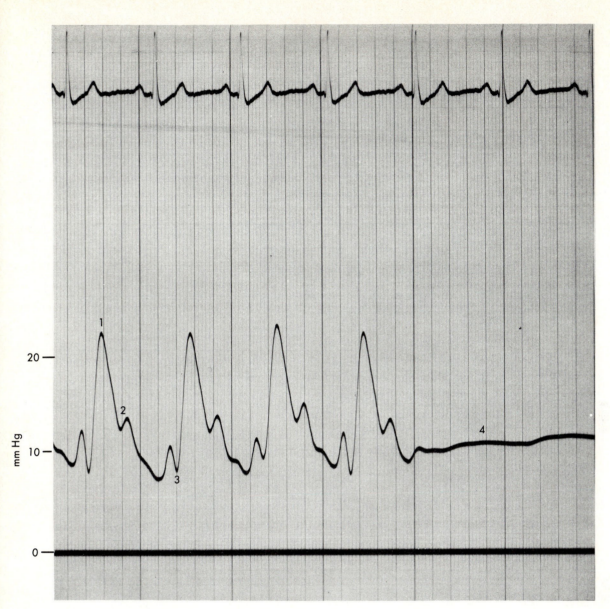

ANALYSIS

Rhythm:

Pressure(s):

Waveform characteristics and measurements:

1. _____ ; _____ mm Hg

2. _____ ; _____ mm Hg

3. _____ ; _____ mm Hg

4. _____ ; _____ mm Hg

5. _____ ; _____ mm Hg

6. _____ ; _____ mm Hg

7. _____ ; _____ mm Hg

Suspected abnormality:

Comments:

ANALYSIS

Rhythm: NSR

Pressure(s): PA

Waveform characteristics and measurements:

1.	PA systolic	;	24 mm Hg
2.	Dicrotic notch	;	mm Hg
3.	PA end-diastolic	;	10 mm Hg
4.	PA electrical mean	;	12 mm Hg
5.		;	mm Hg
6.		;	mm Hg
7.		;	mm Hg

Suspected abnormality: Normal

Comments:

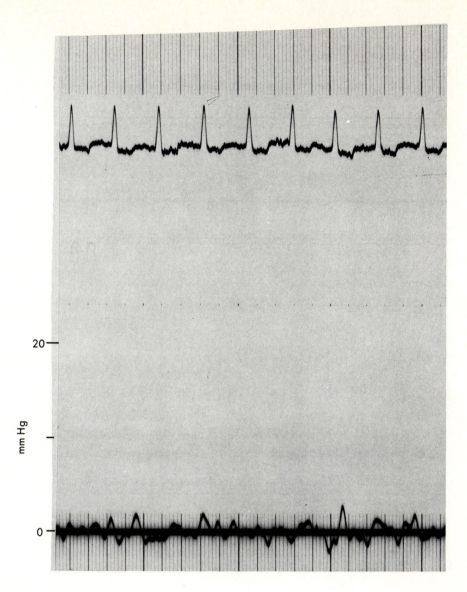

ANALYSIS

Rhythm:

Pressure(s):

Waveform characteristics and measurements:

1. _____ ; _____ mm Hg

2. _____ ; _____ mm Hg

3. _____ ; _____ mm Hg

4. _____ ; _____ mm Hg

5. _____ ; _____ mm Hg

6. _____ ; _____ mm Hg

7. _____ ; _____ mm Hg

Suspected abnormality:

Comments:

ANALYSIS

Rhythm: NSR

Pressure(s): RA

Waveform characteristics and measurements:

1. _____Mean_____ ; _____0_____ mm Hg

2. _____ ; _____ mm Hg

3. _____ ; _____ mm Hg

4. _____ ; _____ mm Hg

5. _____ ; _____ mm Hg

6. _____ ; _____ mm Hg

7. _____ ; _____ mm Hg

Suspected abnormality:

Comments: This pressure waveform is abnormally low due to incorrect placement of the transducer air reference above the level of the right atrium, or incorrect scale selection.

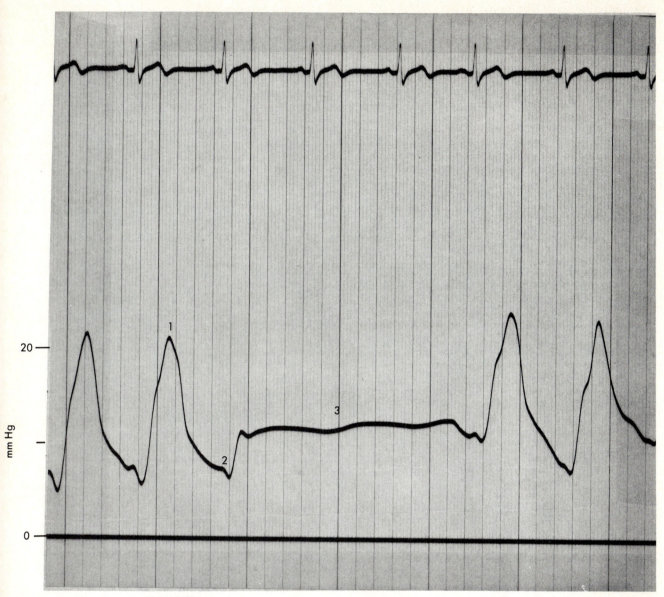

ANALYSIS

Rhythm:

Pressure(s):

Waveform characteristics and measurements:

1. _____ ; _____ mm Hg
2. _____ ; _____ mm Hg
3. _____ ; _____ mm Hg
4. _____ ; _____ mm Hg
5. _____ ; _____ mm Hg
6. _____ ; _____ mm Hg
7. _____ ; _____ mm Hg

Suspected abnormality:

Comments:

ANALYSIS

Rhythm: NSR

Pressure(s): PA

Waveform characteristics and measurements:

1.	PA systolic	;	22	mm Hg
2.	PA end-diastolic	;	7	mm Hg
3.	PA electrical mean	;	12	mm Hg
4.		;		mm Hg
5.		;		mm Hg
6.		;		mm Hg
7.		;		mm Hg

Suspected abnormality: Damped PA pressure

Comments: The slow upstroke and lack of dicrotic notch on this PA pressure tracing may be due to fibrin at the tip of the catheter, which produces a damped pressure tracing.

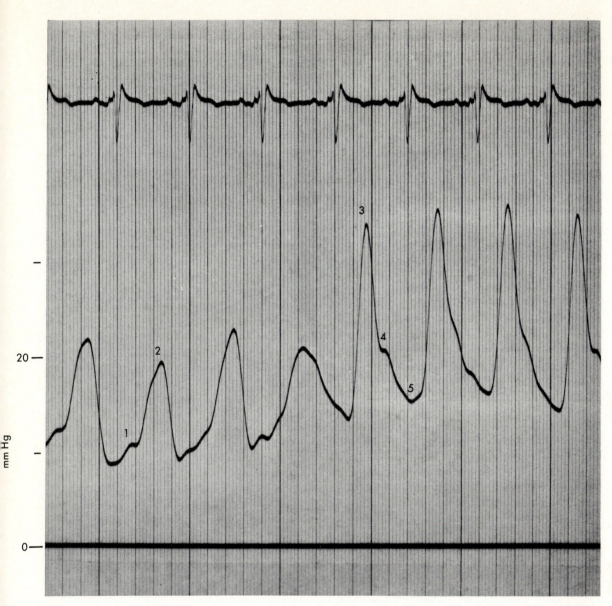

ANALYSIS

Rhythm:

Pressure(s):

Waveform characteristics and measurements:

1. _____ ; _____ mm Hg

2. _____ ; _____ mm Hg

3. _____ ; _____ mm Hg

4. _____ ; _____ mm Hg

5. _____ ; _____ mm Hg

6. _____ ; _____ mm Hg

7. _____ ; _____ mm Hg

Suspected abnormality:

Comments:

ANALYSIS

Rhythm: NSR

Pressure(s): PAW to PA

Waveform characteristics and measurements:

1.	PAW *a* wave	;	12	mm Hg
2.	PAW *v* wave	;	22	mm Hg
3.	PA systolic	;	35	mm Hg
4.	Dicrotic notch	;		mm Hg
5.	PA end-diastolic	;	14	mm Hg
6.		;		mm Hg
7.		;		mm Hg

Suspected abnormality: Mitral regurgitation

Comments: The dominant and elevated PAW *v* wave and rapid *y* descent indicate mitral regurgitation with an increase in LA volume during ventricular systole. The PAW *a* wave is of high normal value. Note the correlation between the PAW *a* wave (12 mm Hg) and the PAedp (14 mm Hg).

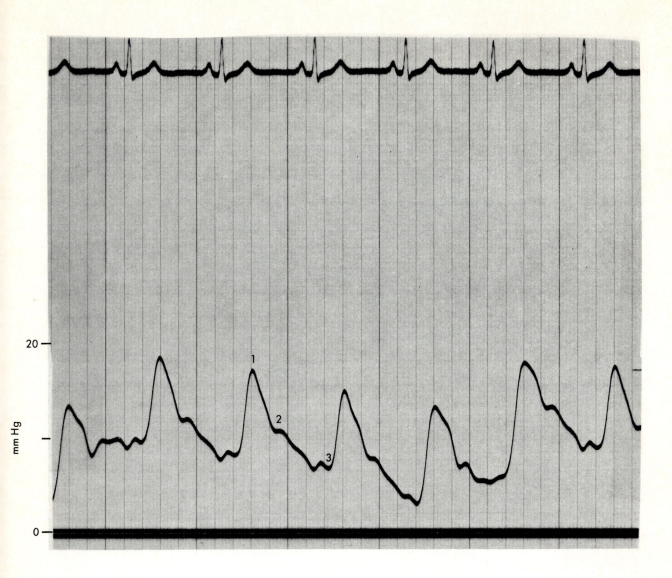

ANALYSIS

Rhythm:

Pressure(s):

Waveform characteristics and measurements:

1. _____ ; _____ mm Hg

2. _____ ; _____ mm Hg

3. _____ ; _____ mm Hg

4. _____ ; _____ mm Hg

5. _____ ; _____ mm Hg

6. _____ ; _____ mm Hg

7. _____ ; _____ mm Hg

Suspected abnormality:

Comments: 273

ANALYSIS

Rhythm: NSR

Pressure(s): PA

Waveform characteristics and measurements:

1. _____ PA systolic _____ ; _____ 18 _____ mm Hg
2. _____ Dicrotic notch _____ ; _____ mm Hg
3. _____ PA end-diastolic _____ ; _____ 8 _____ mm Hg
4. _____ ; _____ mm Hg
5. _____ ; _____ mm Hg
6. _____ ; _____ mm Hg
7. _____ ; _____ mm Hg

Suspected abnormality: Normal

Comments: Note the normal respiratory variation.

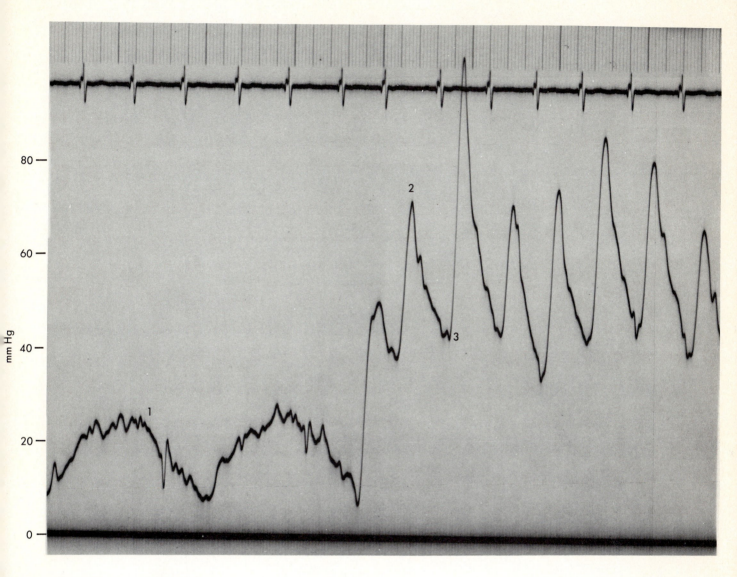

ANALYSIS

Rhythm:

Pressure(s):

Waveform characteristics and measurements:

1. _____ ; _____ mm Hg

2. _____ ; _____ mm Hg

3. _____ ; _____ mm Hg

4. _____ ; _____ mm Hg

5. _____ ; _____ mm Hg

6. _____ ; _____ mm Hg

7. _____ ; _____ mm Hg

Suspected abnormality:

Comments:

ANALYSIS

Rhythm: Atrial fibrillation

Pressure(s): PAW to PA

Waveform characteristics and measurements:

1. _____ PAW mean _____ ; _____ 15 _____ mm Hg
2. _____ PA systolic _____ ; _____ 78 _____ mm Hg
3. _____ PA end-diastolic _____ ; _____ 40 _____ mm Hg
4. _____ ; _____ mm Hg
5. _____ ; _____ mm Hg
6. _____ ; _____ mm Hg
7. _____ ; _____ mm Hg

Suspected abnormality: Primary pulmonary hypertension

Comments: The rapid ventricular rate, the respiratory variation, and the fibrillatory waves in the PAW pressure make identification of the v wave difficult. For this reason the mean PAW pressure is used to reflect LVedp. Note the marked disparity between the PAW mean pressure (15 mm Hg) and the PAedp (40 mm Hg). This is due to primary pulmonary vascular disease and elevated PVR. In this situation only the PAW pressure can be used as a reflection of LVedp.

Bibliography

Alpert, J.S.: Hemodynamic monitoring: the basics, Primary Cardiol., May 1981, pp. 113-126.

Daily, E.K., and Schroeder, J.S.: Techniques in bedside hemodynamic monitoring, St. Louis, 1980, The C.V. Mosby Co.

Forrester, J.S., Diamond, G., and Swan, H.J.: Bedside diagnosis of latent cardiac complications in acutely ill patients, J.A.M.A. **226:**60-61, 1973.

Gorlin, R.: Practical cardiac hemodynamics, N. Engl. J. Med. **296:**203-205, 1977.

Grossman, W.: Cardiac catheterization and angiography, Philadelphia, 1980, Lea & Febiger.

Hancock, E.W.: On the elastic and rigid forms of constrictive pericarditis, Am. Heart J. **100:**917-923, 1980.

Kelman, G.R.: Applied cardiovascular physiology, Boston, 1979, Butterworths Inc.

King, E.D.: Influence of mechanical ventilation and pulmonary disease on pulmonary artery pressure monitoring, C.M.A. J. **121:**901-904, 1979.

Lorell, M.: Right ventricular infarction: clinical diagnosis and differentiation from cardiac tamponade and pericardial constriction, Am. J. Cardiol. **43:**465-471, 1979.

Understanding hemodynamic measurements made with the Swan-Ganz catheter, Santa Ana, Calif., 1979, Edwards Laboratories.